T0177889

Caring for the Family Caregiver

Caring for the Family Caregiver

*Palliative Care Communication
and Health Literacy*

ELAINE WITTENBERG, PHD

ASSOCIATE PROFESSOR
COMMUNICATION STUDIES
CALIFORNIA STATE UNIVERSITY LOS ANGELES
LOS ANGELES, CA

JOY V. GOLDSMITH, PHD

PROFESSOR, HEALTH COMMUNICATION
COMMUNICATION AND FILM
UNIVERSITY OF MEMPHIS
MEMPHIS, TN

SANDRA L. RAGAN, PHD

PROFESSOR EMERITA
DEPARTMENT OF COMMUNICATION
UNIVERSITY OF OKLAHOMA
NORMAN, OK

TERRI ANN PARNELL, DNP, MA, RN, FAAN

PRINCIPAL & FOUNDER
HEALTH LITERACY PARTNERS, LLC
GARDEN CITY, NY

OXFORD
UNIVERSITY PRESS

OXFORD
UNIVERSITY PRESS

Oxford University Press is a department of the University of Oxford. It furthers
the University's objective of excellence in research, scholarship, and education
by publishing worldwide. Oxford is a registered trade mark of Oxford University
Press in the UK and certain other countries.

Published in the United States of America by Oxford University Press
198 Madison Avenue, New York, NY 10016, United States of America.

© Oxford University Press 2021

All rights reserved. No part of this publication may be reproduced, stored in
a retrieval system, or transmitted, in any form or by any means, without the
prior permission in writing of Oxford University Press, or as expressly permitted
by law, by license, or under terms agreed with the appropriate reproduction
rights organization. Inquiries concerning reproduction outside the scope of the
above should be sent to the Rights Department, Oxford University Press, at the
address above.

You must not circulate this work in any other form
and you must impose this same condition on any acquirer.

Library of Congress Cataloging-in-Publication Data
Names: Wittenberg, Elaine, author. | Goldsmith, Joy V., author. | Ragan, Sandra L., author. |
Parnell, Terri Ann, author.
Title: Caring for the family caregiver : palliative care communication and health literacy /
Elaine Wittenberg, Joy V. Goldsmith, Sandra L. Ragan, and Terri Ann Parnell.
Description: New York, NY : Oxford University Press, 2021. |
Includes bibliographical references and index. Identifiers: LCCN 2020014212 (print) |
LCCN 2020014213 (ebook) | ISBN 9780190055233 (paperback) |
ISBN 9780190055257 (epub) | ISBN 9780190055264 (online)
Subjects: MESH: Caregivers | Palliative Care | Communication |
Health Literacy Classification: LCC R726.8 (print) |
LCC R726.8 (ebook) | NLM WY 200 | DDC 616.02/9—dc23
LC record available at https://lccn.loc.gov/2020014212
LC ebook record available at https://lccn.loc.gov/2020014213

This material is not intended to be, and should not be considered, a substitute for medical or other
professional advice. Treatment for the conditions described in this material is highly dependent on
the individual circumstances. And, while this material is designed to offer accurate information with
respect to the subject matter covered and to be current as of the time it was written, research and
knowledge about medical and health issues is constantly evolving and dose schedules for medications
are being revised continually, with new side effects recognized and accounted for regularly. Readers
must therefore always check the product information and clinical procedures with the most up-to-date
published product information and data sheets provided by the manufacturers and the most recent
codes of conduct and safety regulation. The publisher and the authors make no representations or
warranties to readers, express or implied, as to the accuracy or completeness of this material. Without
limiting the foregoing, the publisher and the authors make no representations or warranties as to the
accuracy or efficacy of the drug dosages mentioned in the material. The authors and the publisher do
not accept, and expressly disclaim, any responsibility for any liability, loss, or risk that may be claimed
or incurred as a consequence of the use and/or application of any of the contents of this material.

9 8 7 6 5 4 3 2 1
Printed by Marquis, Canada

CONTENTS

By Debra Parker Oliver

An article in the *Huffington Post* with the headline "Who Gives a Rat's Ass About Family Caregivers" says it all (Brenoff, 2016). The article estimated at the time that there were 34 million caregivers in the United States who were saving the country $500 billion. Depending on the source, these numbers may vary, but the consistent facts remain: First, there are a staggering number of family members who are sacrificing their physical health, finances, and careers to care for a family member. Second, there is a personal cost to individuals providing this care. Studies consistently find that family caregivers have more chronic diseases and a higher mortality rate than those who are not caregivers (Bevans & Sternberg, 2012; Oliver et al., 2017; Stenberg et al., 2010). Finally, despite the emotional and physical strain experienced by caregivers, healthcare providers fail to consider them as partners with the healthcare team.

A study of family caregivers of palliative care patients in Malaysia articulated the suffering of caregivers in a systematic way. Interviewing caregivers of patients enrolled in palliative care, they found common experiences they describe as *interactional suffering* (Beng et al., 2014). This term describes the suffering of caregivers of patients with serious illness, experienced in interactions with healthcare providers. From their interviews they created a conceptual model to help understand the caregiving experience. They categorized the narratives into five themes, which included issues with attention, understanding, communication, competence, and limitation. At the heart of all interactional suffering themes were communication issues between the healthcare team and the caregivers. Most of the suffering was unnecessary and possibly avoidable if the healthcare providers acknowledged their treatment of serious illness as a "family disease" and had the tools necessary to improve communication with the family. This study, like the cases presented in this book, demonstrates the need for family-centered care and family-centered communication, not only in palliative care, but in healthcare in general.

Caring for the Family Caregiver is an extensive practical tool kit for healthcare providers across the healthcare continuum. Regardless if it is a mother caring for a child with a developmental disability, a wife caring for a husband with a long-term chronic illness, or a daughter sitting at the bedside of her father who is enrolled in hospice, family caregivers are the silent "other patient" in the healthcare drama. Healthcare providers who do not attend to the needs of the caregiver not only inflict interactional suffering, but also dilute their treatment by not engaging the caregiver as a partner. In fact, they may unintentionally do harm as the caregiver flounders and thus patient treatment fails. As noted by one dying cancer patient in an educational YouTube video of his cancer journey, "There are two patients not one" (Video 28: https://legaciesfromthelivingroom.com/oliver-videos/).

If we are to eliminate the interactional suffering experienced by family caregivers, we must train both the caregiver and the healthcare team for the important interaction and roles that are required for the successful care of the patient. Caregivers lack information, skills, and emotional support for the tireless task they are volunteering for. They need to be taught how to advocate for themselves and their patients and how to best communicate with the healthcare team. Likewise, healthcare providers have the skills and knowledge to provide outstanding patient-centered care; however, they are not taught the importance of the family caregiver, nor do they always understand that experience or how to help.

Caring for the Family Caregiver uses an extensive literature review to highlight the challenges facing family caregivers. Using a pragmatic approach and integrating the science with real-world narratives, the text brings the literature to life, allowing a systematic approach for providers to understand the lived caregiving experience. Finally, the book provides methods to assess family caregiver needs and more effectively address them. These tools get to the heart of addressing interactional suffering by offering providers concrete actions not only for assessment but also for behavioral change. This unique volume fills a critical gap in a healthcare team's training. This knowledge and set of tools have the potential not only to make real change in interactions with family caregivers but also to create a healthcare system that is family centered. Exemplifying the philosophy that there are two patients in the healthcare drama, not just the one with the disease, this resource will be invaluable to healthcare providers of any discipline or role. This is the first step in eliminating the interactional suffering experienced by family caregivers.

Debra Parker Oliver, PhD, MSW
Paul Revere Family Professor of Family Medicine
University of Missouri
Columbia, Missouri

Caring for the Family Caregiver is the culmination to date of our 15-plus-year quest to make visible the intersections of palliative care communication with the care of patients experiencing chronic and/or terminal illness. In this journey, we have discussed why palliative care is rooted in communication and narrative (Ragan et al., 2008); derived a model represented by the acronym COMFORT that details multiple communication facets of palliative care (Wittenberg-Lyles et al., 2013); studied three family caregiver illness journeys for palliative care and the subsequent patient/caregiver ramifications (Wittenberg-Lyles et al., 2011); and have discovered a family caregiver typology identifying four distinctive kinds of caregiving, referred to as the Family Caregiver Communication Typology (FCCT; Wittenberg-Lyles et al., 2012).

The FCCT was originally developed as a practice approach for the COMFORT model. The acronym COMFORT represents the seven basic principles of palliative care communication; C–connect, O–options, M–make meaning, F–family caregivers, O–openings, R–relating, and T–team. The *F* in COMFORT, family caregivers, includes communication strategies for tailoring communication to better meet the needs of each caregiver type. Over the last eight years, the FCCT has been introduced and validated by more than 10,000 healthcare providers nationally (Wittenberg et al., 2016, 2018).

The FCCT provides a way to measure communication characteristics by assessing caregiver challenges when finding information, talking about illness, and learning how to work with healthcare providers. Inherently embedded within the family system, these characteristics help inform healthcare providers with ways to enhance caregiver health literacy and foster communication needs and preferences. We believe that the clinical application of the FCCT, as manifested by research with patients, family caregivers, and providers, is clinically relevant and essential when caring for the family caregiver.

Our initial efforts to learn more about the family system revealed that families had difficulty adjusting to illness and that this adjustment was as much about adjusting as a family as it was about adjusting to the impending loss and changing identity of a family member. Recognizing that each person within the same family has a unique family experience, we turned to family communication patterns to explore the strain wrought by chronic or terminal illness. The heightened burden and difficulties that families experience while continuing with their day-to-day functioning and activities of daily living, tremendously affect medical, financial, and social decisions that now need to be made. We learned that the act of caregiving—the medical and nursing skills that are suddenly critical—is just one small part of the caregiving equation. Additionally, we discovered that communication and health literacy challenges embedded in the caregiving role are significant stressors. And, most important, we posited that palliative care, because it recognizes and addresses these stressors among caregivers, is the overarching perspective that should be adopted in caring for the family caregiver.

In this volume, we again detail a palliative care approach to patient caregiving, addressing the challenges and strategies for meeting the communication and health literacy needs of family caregivers to ensure a "comforted journey" for the patient, where palliative care is embraced early in the disease course and eventually culminates in hospice care. A comforted journey is dependent upon *open awareness*—communication that ensures that discussions about the disease trajectory and end of life planning are part of chronic illness care (Glaser & Strauss, 1967). A guiding principle of FCCT is that all family caregivers have unique health literacy needs, based upon previous family expectations, roles, responsibilities, spiritual or cultural preferences, and decision-making patterns, and each caregiver needs education and support for communicating with the patient, family, and healthcare providers about illness. Ideally, this education and support should come at the initial point of diagnosis and continue throughout the disease trajectory. Psychosocial and family support includes open communication about advance care planning and end-of-life discussions, addressing mental health difficulties, caregiver interventions focused on self-care, connecting caregivers to community resources, addressing anticipatory grief, family meetings to discuss complicated interpersonal dynamics, and discussions about spiritual and cultural beliefs (Farabelli et al., 2020). This book is designed to meet the needs of healthcare providers and students across a variety of palliative care and chronic illness disciplines.

For this volume, we are fortunate to have access to an abundance of family caregivers from which we gathered family experiences about living with a chronic illness diagnosis. It is from the many families and their approaches to and stories about illness that we derive the design for this volume as well as the proposed pathway for improving chronic illness care. Participants come from clinical and nonclinical settings. City of Hope Medical Center and Markey Cancer Center served as sites for cancer family caregiver stories and support group data. Caregiver focus groups held across the country provided oncology-specific feedback about caregiver needs and desires in the caregiving journey. Interviews with caregivers of family members with type 2 diabetes, chronic obstructive pulmonary disease, cancer, or Alzheimer's disease across a variety of ethnically and culturally diverse community settings, provided rich, nonclinical descriptive data about family experiences, and caregiving. A social support agency in the mid-South allowed us to have access to HIV caregivers who described their challenges in helping care recipients stay in care. Additionally, collections of public domain websites that feature family caregivers also provided further narrative articulations of family and chronic illness. All references to specific individuals have been changed.

As we came to understand the stories and experiences of our participants in their various journeys, we wished to represent in detail the four family caregiver communication types, the Manager, Partner, Carrier, and Lone caregivers, as each of them vary in their communication and health literacy abilities. The design of this volume is based on these families, their disease journeys, and their stories. Our hope is that this volume will be used as a guidebook and be adapted for future interventions aimed at skill building for caregivers. We are so grateful to those family caregivers who were willing to trust us enough to share their illness narratives.

Book cover and chapter illustrations provided by Carol Aust from Oakland, California.

REFERENCES

Beng, T. S., Guan, N. C., Jane, L. E., & Chin, L. E. (2014, May). Health care interactional suffering in palliative care. *American Journal of Hospice & Palliative Medicine*, *31*(3), 307–314. https://doi.org/10.1177/1049909113490065

Bevans, M., & Sternberg, E. M. (2012). Caregiving burden, stress, and health effects among family caregivers of adult cancer patients. *JAMA*, *307*(4), 398–403. https://doi.org/10.1001/jama.2012.29

Brenoff, A. (2016, September 1). No one gives a rat's ass about family caregivers. *Huffington Post*. Retrieved from https://www.huffpost.com/entry/no-one-gives-a-rats-ass-about-family-caregivers_n_57bc8c36e4b0b51733a61582

Farabelli, J. P., Kimberly, S. M., Altilio, T., Otis-Green, S., Dale, H., Dombrowski, D., . . . Jones, C. A. (2020). Top ten tips palliative care clinicians should know about psychosocial and family support. *Journal of Palliative Medicine*, *23*(2), 280–286. https://doi.org/10.1089/jpm.2019.0506

Glaser, B., & Strauss, A. (1967). *The discovery of grounded theory: Strategies for qualitative research*. Chicago, IL: Aldine.

Oliver, D. P., Demiris, G., Washington, K. T., Clark, C., & Thomas-Jones, D. (2017). Challenges and strategies for hospice caregivers: A qualitative analysis. *Gerontologist*, *57*(4), 648–656. https://doi.org/10.1093/geront/gnw054

Ragan, S., Wittenberg-Lyles, E., Goldsmith, J., & Sanchez-Reilly, S. (2008). *Communication as comfort: Multiple voices in palliative care*. New York, NY: Routledge, Taylor and Francis.

Stenberg, U., Ruland, C. M., & Miaskowski, C. (2010). Review of the literature on the effects of caring for a patient with cancer. *Psycho-Oncology*, *19*(10), 1013–1025. https://doi.org/10.1002/pon.1670

Wittenberg, E., Ferrell, B., Goldsmith, J., Ragan, S. L., & Buller, H. (2018). COMFORT™(SM) communication for oncology nurses: Program overview and preliminary evaluation of a nationwide train-the-trainer course. *Patient Education and Counseling, 101*(3), 467–474. https://doi.org/10.1016/j.pec.2017.09.012

Wittenberg, E., Ferrell, B., Goldsmith, J., Ragan, S. L., & Paice, J. (2016). Assessment of a statewide palliative care team training course: COMFORT Communication for Palliative Care Teams. *Journal of Palliative Medicine, 19*(7), 746–752. doi:10.1089/jpm.2015.0552

Wittenberg-Lyles, E., Goldsmith, J., Ferrell, B., & Ragan, S. L. (2013). *Communication in Palliative Nursing.* New York, NY; Oxford University Press.

Wittenberg-Lyles, E., Goldsmith, J., Demiris, G., Oliver, D. P., & Stone, J. (2012, Jan). The Impact of Family Communication Patterns on Hospice Family Caregivers: A New Typology. *Journal of Hospice & Palliative Nursing, 14*(1), 25–33. https://doi.org/10.1097/NJH.0b013e318233114b

Wittenberg-Lyles, E., Goldsmith, J., & Ragan, S. (2011, Jun 1). The shift to early palliative care: a typology of illness journeys and the role of nursing. *Clinical Journal of Oncology Nursing, 15*(3), 304–310. https://doi.org/10.1188/11.CJON.304-310

The Family Caregiving Imperative

As we write, four dear friends suffer from chronic, perhaps terminal disease, and all have been confounded by the difficulties of navigating the healthcare system. Their stories have left us feeling almost useless as scholars and clinicians of palliative care communication and family caregiving: What can we write that will help those with serious illness and the people who love them better plan their disease journeys? How can listening to their stories affect any change in their treatment decisions? While we are devoting an entire chapter of the current volume to health literacy, one of our primary theoretical foundations, the illness stories we have heard belie an easy answer to developing and utilizing an informed knowledge of healthcare, even when the ill and their caregivers have advanced degrees.

In a particularly frustrating instance, a wife was striving to determine whether her husband, newly diagnosed with dementia Lewy body, would benefit from enrolling in a clinical trial that had been recommended by his neurologist. Knowing of our expertise, she forwarded the description of the clinical trial and the informed consent form. But none of us could decipher which prescription drugs were excluded from the trial: her husband was doing well on a current antidepressant, but if he had to stop taking the drug during the four months of the trial, would potential benefits from it outweigh the risk of his possibly being severely depressed? Further, the nurse assigned to oversee the administration of the trial wasn't able to answer her question about whether the drug was precluded. How can a person be expected to make an informed decision about treatment options when there's no clarity in the written or spoken word by those involved with administering the trial?

Additional stories revealed the frustration of family caregivers attempting to understand and to carry out medical procedures at home: two adult sons of a friend who underwent surgery for non-Hodgkin's lymphoma in her tibia were not given clear or sufficient information about how to relieve her postsurgical pain after she was prematurely discharged from the hospital. The husband of another friend whose wife is suffering from stage 3 ovarian cancer did not get written instructions about obtaining a prescription for steroids following her first chemotherapy induction: as a result, she suffered needlessly without the drug that would have alleviated some of the severe side effects of the chemotherapy.

Yet sharing and hearing these stories is vital to our understanding of how communication directly impacts our treatment choices, our pain levels, and our overall peace of mind that we are receiving optimal care in one of the world's wealthiest and most health-knowledgeable nations. The stories also manifest our complete reliance on the health literacy skills, perseverance, and resilience of family caregivers, even when they are exhausted by and distraught over their loved ones' illnesses. The family caregiver is the backbone of the nation's long-term care system. The labors of caregiving are dynamic as the nature and extent of care are constantly moving targets (Milliken et al., 2019). A caregiver is an unpaid person (like a partner, a child, a neighbor, a friend, a family member) central to assisting a care recipient with the activities of daily living and/or health-care labors. This kind of person is very different than a paid and formally trained healthcare provider who provides support and care in the home or a care set-ting outside of the home. Originally coined "informal caregiver" in the 1980s, suggesting "casual, unstructured, unofficial care—pleasant but not essential," we surmise that caregivers would find this term invalidating as there is unquestion-ingly nothing "informal" or unessential about the care they provide (Stall et al., 2019). Still, the reality is that many caregivers often don't recognize themselves in a caregiving role even when they are deeply into it and are tremendously impacted by their caregiving responsibilities. And when illness is chronic, the prospect of a constant, unabating, ceaseless level of care and resources can be depleting for a family caregiver.

CHRONIC ILLNESS: THE INCREASING DEMAND ON FAMILY CAREGIVING

The distinct spectrum of chronic disease is replacing infectious disease as the leading cause of morbidity in the world today. The Institute of Health Metrics and Evaluation identifies noncommunicable illness including coronary heart dis-ease, stroke, diabetes mellitus type 2, neurogenerative diseases, and renal failure as the cause behind 72% of deaths in 2018 (Friedman et al., 2016). The World Health Organization identified chronic disease as the leading cause of death and disability worldwide. This global pandemic of chronic disease has emerged at the same time that the world birth rate exceeds the death rate, increasing the number of living people on the planet. At the same time, people are living longer except in the United States where longevity is decreasing!. In developing nations, the aging and elderly populations are increasing significantly because of these anthropo-logical changes in human life and development (WHO CVD Risk Chart Working Group, 2019). The World Populations Prospects released by the United Nations in 2019 estimated the number of people in the world at 7.55 billion human beings. The same study, using projections of current birth and death rates, estimates that this number will increase to 9 billion by 2040 (United Nations, 2019).

More than 160 million Americans live with at least one chronic illness, and 7 out of 10 Americans die from chronic disease (Torres et al., 2017). Twenty percent of the United States' population will be 65 years and older by 2030. The majority of adults will develop or contract one or more chronic illnesses in the latter third of their lives. They will live protractedly with illness for years before death. More often than not, these years of illness are framed by increasing functional dependence and frailty, increasing family support needs, and increasing physical and psychological discomfort (Wittenberg-Lyles et al., 2011). Of the top 10 causes of death in 2015, the top 2 were chronic illnesses (heart disease and cancer), and 6 (heart disease, cancer, respiratory disease, diabetes, Alzheimer's disease, kidney disease) of the 10 causes were chronic illnesses, with Alzheimer's disease more than doubling in its number of deaths between 2010 and 2015 (Aldridge & Bradley, 2017). This description, however, suggests a simplicity in these diagnoses, when in reality multimorbidity (having two or more chronic conditions) is increasingly common. Current epidemiology projections estimate that the number of Americans with multimorbidities will increase by 30% between 2000 and 2030 (Aldridge & Bradley, 2017).

For those dying from chronic illness, there was no increase in the numbers of those receiving end-of-life care or those dying at home between 2010 and 2015. This is of concern in light of the increasing numbers of death from chronic illness (Sathitratanacheewin et al., 2018).

Despite a 2015 Institute of Medicine Report that emphasized the need for improving end-of-life care and palliative care services, so many people still die in hospital locations that they would not choose (Institute of Medicine, 2015). Recent research identifies predictors of death in the hospital, including those patients who tend to be younger, with multimorbidities, suffering from cancer or dementia, and who had received less care in outpatient visits (Hicks et al., 2018).

Chronic conditions are defined by the World Health Organization (Ashida, Marcum, & Koehly, 2017) as requiring "ongoing management over a period of years or decades" and cover a wide range of health problems such as heart disease, diabetes, asthma, HIV/AIDS, depression, and schizophrenia. Many conditions previously categorized as rapidly progressing terminal conditions have evolved into chronic health illnesses that patients will live with for years. Caregiving for someone with multimorbidities is exponentially complicated by compounded medication management, coordination of providers from an array of specialties, and prioritizing goals of care.

A Population at Risk

(From a cancer caregiver support group)

> CAREGIVER 1: I've cancelled all of mine [healthcare appointments] mainly because she was in the, ya know, she was at the time I had several of them but she was really sick with the transplant and I haven't rescheduled yet. It's just kind of crazy with going there to the city Monday, and then

Tuesdays and Thursdays the nurses and PT comes and home health nurse
comes. It's kind of hard—
NURSE: Hard to fit it in.
SOCIAL WORKER: It is.
CAREGIVER 2: Well this is xxx and I took care of my mother last year and
cancelled my appointments last year and then this year with my husband
being sick I haven't made any appointments so . . .

About one in six Americans (adult aged, as there are no reliable numbers on
caregivers under the age of 18) provide an estimated 37 billion hours of unpaid
care to family or friends, with an estimated value of $470 billion in 2013, up from
$450 billion in 2009 (AARP Public Policy Institute et al., 2015). This population of
caregivers is not prepared to fill the demanding needs of a care recipient with little
support and while also suffering themselves from poor health and unaddressed
healthcare needs. Increasing cuts to the amount of funded hospital care, limited discharge planning/resources, and growing medical advances apply more pressure to
caregivers who are shouldering care burden (amount of time spent giving care) for
extended periods of time. These caregivers themselves have less health insurance
coverage as a result of time out of the workforce. Research in the last two decades
has consistently found that caregivers suffer from higher levels of depression and
other mental health illnesses than the non-caregiving population. Depressed
caregivers are more likely themselves to have substance abuse or dependence and
chronic disease as well. Over half of caregivers report a chronic condition, nearly
twice the rate of non-caregivers (National Alliance for Caregiving, 2018).

The average caregiver age is 49, with caregivers between 18 and 49 years accounting for 48% of the caregiver population and those over 65 years accounting
for 34% (National Alliance for Caregiving and AARP, 2015). Older caregivers
are more likely to care for a spouse or partner, with the time spent caregiving
increasing as the caregiver's age increases.

Around 75% of all caregivers are female who may spend up to 50% more time caregiving than males, with males providing less personal care than females (Institute
on Aging, 2019). Their lives are impacted more negatively than male caregivers, as
they report higher levels of depression, anxiety, and lower levels of physical health
and happiness than males. Mental health challenges increase for those women providing care more than 36 hours a week (Family Caregiver Alliance, 2019).

In 2015, almost 10% of caregivers identified as LGBTQ+. Hours of care from
this population is similar by gender (26 hours for men vs. 28 hours for women
per week). As the LGBTQ+ population is predicted to double from 9% to 20% in
the next two decades, it is important to note that as a population they are twice as
likely to age as a single person and to reside alone; they are four times as likely not
to have children (Espinoza, 2014).

Hispanics have the highest rate of caregivers across racial/ethnic groups (21%),
followed by African American caregivers (20.3%), Asian American caregivers
(19.7%), and White caregivers (16.9%). Their rate of caregiving correlates with
their progression of age, with Hispanic caregivers averaging 42.7 years, African

American caregivers averaging 44.2 years, Asian Americans averaging 46.6 years, and White caregivers averaging 52.5 years of age. Similarly, Hispanic and African American caregivers experience highest burden at 30 hours of care per week, followed by White caregivers at 20 hours per week and then Asian Americans at 16 hours per week (National Alliance for Caregiving and AARP, 2015).

Without question, caregiving is now known to have harmful effects on a caregiver's mental and physical health. Caregiver health declines during the period of caregiving, and those caring for a spouse are most likely to experience poor health due to the intensity and unrelenting nature of spousal responsibility (National Alliance for Caregiving and AARP, 2015). The following caregivers rated their physical strain as highest: those providing care for more than a year, older caregivers; those with high burden, dementia caregivers; and those living with the care recipient. The greater the number of activities of daily living performed is proportional to the deterioration of physical health for the caregiver (National Alliance for Caregiving and AARP, 2015). The negative emotional and physical effects of caregiving are the greatest for caregivers aged 18 to 29. A correlation exists between caregiver income and the state of their own health, with caregivers earning the least experiencing the greatest personal health challenges (National Alliance for Caregiving and AARP, 2015).

Most caregivers have symptoms of depression. Caregivers are at particular risk for cardiovascular syndromes like high blood pressure or heart disease, with poor self-care and stressful conditions putting them at a twofold increased risk for such maladies (National Alliance for Caregiving and AARP, 2015). Smoking rates and poor eating are more common for caregivers, and the likelihood not to fill prescriptions for their own care because of cost is much higher than in the non-caregiving population (National Alliance for Caregiving, 2018, January). It is well established that caregivers do not have time to prepare meals or to exercise (Reinhard et al., 2019). Strongly established, caregiving is related to increased mortality; caregivers pay the ultimate price (Family Caregiver Alliance, 2006), dying more quickly than non-caregivers and living less well and often in states of poorer health.

Most caregivers live within 20 minutes of the care recipient. This figure has steadily increased over the last 10 years. About 30% of all caregivers are long-distance caregivers (LDC). The LDCs have the highest caregiving expenses, and they reside an average of seven hours travel time away from the care recipient. These caregivers are more likely to report emotional distress (Cagle & Munn, 2012) than those living nearby.

A total of 5.5 million caregivers are caring for former or current military personnel in the United States. Nine out of 10 of these caregivers are women and provide care for more than 10 years. These caregivers report highest anxiety, stress, and sleep deprivation; are most likely to be employed; are younger than the larger caregiver populations; and tend to care for a recipient with multiple behavioral health needs (Ramchand et al., 2014).

(Ms. Paulette, a spousal cancer caregiver for 20 years)
"I know one thing—taking care of sick people will kill you."

Children and Youth Caregivers

As invisible as the caregiver can be in the healthcare world, children who serve as caregivers are the most painfully invisible caregivers in systems of care. Youth as young as 8, 9, and 10 years of age are partially or completely responsible for the caregiving of a parent, grandparent, sibling, or other family member. Shopping, cooking, cleaning, and bathing can fall to children in households that have no other care support. In the midst of school, homework, and activities, caregiving displaces age appropriate involvements such as friendships, playing, imagining, receiving care, and learning—all essential and well-recognized as important to the development of healthy and productive children (Coller & Kuo, 2016).

It seemed like Ginny always had Kate, aged 12, in tow because Ginny was the grandma, and that's what grandmas do. As the months passed in learning more about my neighbors, the complexity of the chronic illnesses in that household ballooned. Once I was finally inside their home, I could see that Ginny was actually unable to walk. It was so well disguised in the context of her car and her kitchen. I had noticed the scooter on the back of the car and the ramp up to the side door of the kitchen, but also noticed the bustle of errands and shopping. Ginny was administering all cooking and organizational labors from a rolling office chair in the kitchen. She never walked. Kate had become her legs and supplied all movement. When another layer of privacy was peeled back, I eventually saw the sewing room where Ginny was when she wasn't in the kitchen. She sat in a recliner at the sewing machine, working on small projects and fixes. This recliner also served as her bed. It was lined with an absorbent pad. Ginny was incontinent. Kate would change the pad, wash Ginny's soiled clothes, and clean up her waste from the floor when there were bathroom accidents. Ginny suffered from renal failure, type 2 diabetes, was morbidly obese, and had chronic kidney and bladder infections. Her low heart function and dangerously high weight made knee replacement impossible. Over time, her mobility had dwindled. Kate solved these mobility issues whenever they ran errands or navigated tasks inside the house. Kate was making the household possible—at age 12.

Statistics on the number of youth serving as caregivers are unknown. The most published stats estimate that 1.4 million children ages 8 to 18 are serving as caregivers in the United States. This at-risk group is particularly hard to study, identify, and assist because of their age; the adults surrounding them protect access to their experience. Children undertake significant caring roles for relatives or household members who need help resulting from mental illness, aging, disability, and other chronic health conditions with demands that are not appropriate to their age (Brody, 2016).

So many of this invisible group of caregivers come from single-parent/no-parent, low-income households. The most measurable point of deprivation is their academic success. Sleep scarcity and caregiver burden and anxiety fracture academic progress. Few of these caregivers report their caregiving activities and responsibilities and enact a protective pattern of behavior concerning their own labors for the care recipient. Incomplete homework, absenteeism, and poor academic performance are common patterns in this population (Brody, 2016). As more of those facing illness are treated at home, this phenomenon is likely to increase.

Caregiving Tasks: Making the Invisible Visible

(Caregiver in a caregiver support group)

> My son has throat cancer and we're there every day. He takes two treatments every day and he has to take lighter doses because he's had radiation before and I'm there all day every day and live about 30 miles away. So I drive it every day and I have to have him there at 9:00 AM, and then he has another treatment at 3:00. I sit in that lobby every day all day with him.

Maybe it is easy to dismiss what you cannot measure or quantify. As most of the labors of the caregiver unfold in the home, we describe a common list of labors performed by the family caregiver. Thirteen days a month are spent shopping, preparing food, keeping the house livable, doing laundry, transporting the care recipient, and administering medications or executing procedures (catheter, wound cleaning, breathing treatments, etc.). Six days per month are spent on feeding, dressing, grooming, walking, bathing, and toileting. An untold number of hours each month are spent researching care services, disease path information, symptoms/symptom treatments, coordinating provider visits, and navigating financial matters related to care (Family Caregiver Alliance, 2017).

Some caregivers help navigate very complex chronic care for a care recipient. These caregivers may perform medical and nursing tasks and likely assist with activities of daily living like getting in and out of bed, getting dressed, cleaning the patient, helping the patient move in a wheelchair or with a walker. The great secret that we will reveal in this book (hardly a secret to caregivers) is that there is a lot of tasking imposed upon them that they do not like. Caregivers, in many cases, are not happy, want to break free from a family's dependence, and even fantasize and plan to leave their post as caregiver. Some caregivers are pressured to perform the role of caregiver by the care receiver and some by another family member (Reinhard et al., 2019). On average, caregivers spend 25 hours a week providing care, but this number doubles for those caring for a spouse or partner. While the average length of duration for a caregiver role is four years, almost a quarter of all caregivers stay in that role for more than five years, and 15% of caregivers provide care for more than a decade (National Alliance for Caregiving and AARP, 2015).

A majority of caregivers describe playing a highly significant role in monitoring the care recipient's condition and making adjustments to that care, communicating with healthcare professionals and providers on behalf of the patient, and serving as an advocate for the patient with providers, service agencies, and government agencies (National Alliance for Caregiving and AARP, 2015). Four in 10 caregivers are in high burden situations, with 18% in medium burden, and 41% in low burden. Burden of care increases with hours of care provided (AARP Public Policy Institute et al., 2015).

The Financial Cost to Working Caregivers

Most working caregivers feel that they have no choice about taking on caregiving responsibilities, and this sense of obligation is higher for caregivers who provide more than 21 hours of care per week and for live-in caregivers. Most caregivers report having to rearrange their work schedule, decrease their work hours, take unpaid leave, and job loss as a result of caregiving. Caregivers who care for someone with mental or emotional issues report the highest rate of making work accommodations (National Alliance for Caregiving and AARP, 2015). It follows that caregivers' loss of wages, health insurance, retirement savings, and Social Security benefits compound over time and hold serious consequences for the caregiver. Total loss in wages, pensions, retirement funds, and benefits are worse for women, who lose nearly $400,000 due to caregiving compared to men, at $300,000 (MetLife Mature Market Group, 2011). Single females who care for their elderly parents are 2.5 times more likely than non-caregivers to live in poverty in old age (Demitz, 2017). The lower the income and education of a person, the more likely he or she is to be a caregiver (National Alliance for Caregiving and AARP, 2015). The four most common chronic illnesses in the United States today requiring the majority of caregiver hours include dementia, heart disease, cancer, and type 2 diabetes.

DEMENTIA

The care of people with dementia takes place over years and is accomplished primarily by spouses, adult children, and their children's spouses. The majority of these caregivers are women (Alzheimer's Association, 2016). The type of dementia a care recipient presents with influences the level of caregiver burden. Frontotemporal dementia and dementia with Lewy body caregivers produce higher burden ratings compared to Alzheimer's disease caregivers (Svendsboe et al., 2016). Younger caregivers experience higher levels of burden, identified as guilt and anxiety over the impact on their lives. Depression is a significant outcome that is highly predicted by the care recipient's symptoms, being female, and being a spouse of the care recipient. Depressed caregivers of dementia patients have a one in six rate of experiencing suicidal ideation (O'Dwyer et al., 2016).

Physical outcomes for these caregivers, compared to non-caregivers, reveal a higher instance of obesity, cardiovascular disease, and hypertension (Merrilees, 2016). Biomarkers of stress include proteins and hormones that initiate anti-inflammatory responses at a higher rate for dementia caregivers than for non-caregivers. Chromosome components (telomeres) that regulate aging are shorter in caregivers who have delivered care for five years compared with age-matched controls (Damjanovic et al., 2007). Caregivers with coping styles that included distraction and denial experience poorer sleep efficacy than those dementia caregivers whose coping style includes acceptance and problem-solving (Taylor et al., 2015). Most alarming is the sixfold increase in dementia risk for dementia caregivers, a trend that persists even after the death of the care recipient (Dassel et al., 2015).

The interaction shared between the caregiver and recipient has also been shown to impact caregiver outcomes. The closer the dyad, the less depression and higher levels of calm the caregiver experienced (Hsieh et al., 2013). Caregivers interacted less frequently with and offered less support to spouses than non-caregiving spouses. Caregivers with the greatest burden use more negative emotional words than caregivers with less burden or non-caregivers (Ascher et al., 2010). Family communication tensions are understudied to date. However, a study of sibling caregivers revealed that perceived favoritism impacted tensions among siblings, and caregivers who feel other family are not helping enough experience higher caregiver distress (Ashida et al., 2017). Family stressors can translate to interference with decision-making, not sharing labors in the provision of care, and conflict about the progression of the patient's symptoms and their meaning (Suitor et al., 2014).

HEART DISEASE

One in four deaths in the United States, United Kingdom, Canada, and Australia is related to heart disease (Centers for Disease Control, 2019). Chronic obstructive pulmonary disease, congestive heart failure, myocardial infarction, coronary heart disease, and arrhythmia are some of the disorders covered under the umbrella of heart disease. Because symptoms can be so severe and the prognosis poor in advanced cases, some of these specific maladies are treated with palliative care (see more on palliative care in Chapter 3 of this volume). Caregivers of these patients feel overloaded by the burdens of advanced heart disease and want to be acknowledged by healthcare staff in their efforts and concerns (Bangerter et al., 2018).

Heart disease is unique in its symptoms, treatment options, disease trajectories, stigma, and prognosis (Cagle et al., 2017). The greatest need for heart disease caregivers is communication with care providers and healthcare professionals to exchange information about symptoms, pain and symptom management, and disease progression (Wingham et al., 2015). A direct correlation between the provision of inadequate information shared with caregivers and their distress and mental health status has been proven, as well as their increased risk for death compared with caregivers who carried less strain (Sullivan et al., 2016). Substantial evidence identifies heart disease caregivers as having limited understanding about treatments, insufficient support from providers, and scant resources to provide the care needed by the patient at home, as well as spending a great deal of time managing finances for care, arranging/executing transportation for care, and managing the on-site, at home care facility that their house had become (Pressler et al., 2013). Caregivers overseeing heart disease express a uniquely high level of vigilance to perform caregiving tasks correctly but, even more important, to protect patients from performing too many activities and worsening their status. Sustaining these high levels of vigilance over time is directly connected to fatigue and overstimulation of the pituitary adrenal center—both of which are associated with poor health. Changes in the caregiver's relationship with the care recipient over time is also costly to happiness and resilience, underscoring the complexities and effects of communication between caregiver and patient (Sullivan et al., 2016).

CANCER

Cancer caregivers are at increased risk for adverse health effects, morbidity, and mortality. The adverse effects of caregiving include anxiety, depression, physical symptoms, and problems in interpersonal relationships due to social isolation (Moss et al., 2019). Cancer caregivers are expected to be informed and participate in decision-making, keep the care recipient's hope up, support the remaining family, have empathy and be understanding, and share emotions (Reigada et al., 2015). However, caregivers often experience communication apprehension, hesitation to engage in difficult conversations, and a tendency to avoid communication (Wittenberg et al., 2017). Caregivers experience distress from the perceived inability to communicate in difficult situations (Stone et al., 2012). Real or perceived communication challenges impact information needs about treatment, side effects, and how to prepare for managing symptoms at home (Ream et al., 2013).

Role demands and preparedness to manage the caregiving role, ability to maintain self-care, and the emotional response to caregiving contribute to caregiver distress (Fujinami et al., 2015). Family caregivers of persons with cancer experience very high levels of anxiety, even exceeding the anxiety of their loved one (Nipp et al., 2016). In 2018, the National Alliance for Caregiving recognized the need for caregiver support as a national public health issue, recommending caregiver access to comprehensive training to ensure caregivers know how to communicate within the formal healthcare system (National Alliance for Caregiving, 2018).

DIABETES MELLITUS, TYPE 2

Twelve percent of the American population had diabetes in 2015, and 90% of those with the disease suffer from type 2 diabetes mellitus (Wakefield & Vaughan-Sarrazin, 2018). While not always the case, the disease is very often associated with being overweight and leading a sedentary lifestyle. Without good disease management (maintaining a healthy level of blood sugar), this disease can become very complicated for patients to regulate since the disease is closely dependent on meal consumption, physical activity, and medication management. If blood sugars are too high for too long, the small and large blood vessels are damaged, introducing a contagion of complicating events to the life of the care receiver and caregiver.

Cataracts and retinopathy of the eyes can cause loss of vision for the diabetic. Kidney function can be affected through diabetic nephropathy, requiring dialysis or organ transplant. Neuropathy is the damage to all nerves that can occur with high blood sugar levels, but peripheral neuropathy is the most common, impacting the nerves going to the hands and feet. Losing sensation in the feet, in particular, as well as pain, weakness, burning, and tingling are part of this disease process. Diabetics can suffer injury to their feet and not realize it because of neuropathy, causing serious infection that can result in amputation, gangrene, and sepsis (Leontis & Hess-Fischl, 2019).

Caregivers of diabetics predominantly suffer effects from anxiety, depression, and social functioning. Female caregivers report significantly lower scores on mental health measures, and financial concerns were more profound for African American caregivers (Galarraga & Llahan, 2018). When caregivers themselves have a chronic illness or poor family functioning, their mental health and quality of life is lower (Costa & Pereira, 2017). Caregivers of veterans with type 2 diabetes mellitus have higher strain when performing the activities of daily living and receive less help from friends. These caregivers feel somewhat confident in knowing how to help their care recipients, but half of them indicate they had no choice in serving as caregiver (Wakefield & Vaughan-Sarrazin, 2018).

HEALTH LITERACY

Chronic illness should situate the patient and caregiver as one unit of care, prioritizing family communication as a key part of health communication and shared decision-making. Patient and family action upon serious diagnosis is impacted by their individual demographics, health status, previous health knowledge and experience, cultural and spiritual influences, community support, and what is learned from the media/marketplace, or collectively by their health literacy skills (Parnell, 2015). Our current healthcare system is increasingly dependent on patient and family to seek services, carry out treatments, manage chronic and terminal diseases, and effectively communicate to achieve these tasks. While caregivers are involved in decision-making alongside the patient, many report unmet information needs and feeling excluded from the decision-making process (Martin et al., 2019). Essentially, caregiving requires health communication skills for improving healthcare during clinical visits, as well as health literacy skills which involve the ability to obtain, communicate, process, and understand basic health information and services (Office of Disease Prevention and Health Promotion, 2019). We present health literacy and its challenges in Chapter 2.

Caregivers lack information about the help that healthcare professionals can offer, do not always have supportive relationships with providers, and do not always know what to expect (Schulz et al., 2018); they are rarely asked by a healthcare provider about their own needs (Berry et al., 2017). Traditional communication methods between caregivers and healthcare providers, such as clinic visits and phone calls, are not effective in facilitating overall support for caregivers who are often untrained, yet provide unpaid, extensive patient care (Tao et al., 2017). Little is known about differences among caregivers in support service utilization, information needs, and emotional experiences, yet all of these factors contribute to caregiver communication burden and are influenced by health literacy.

Caregiver Communication Burden

(excerpt shared between Dr. Lou/staff and Grace, caregiver of Jensen,
from patient portal)
Per Dr. Lou:
cont:5/30/2019 labs reviewed Dr. Degan
testosterone 139 total(250–827 normal)
HH 11.1/33.1
The anemia had increased since 5/2019 lab results of HH 12.8/37.8
6/28/2019FIt cards-negative and 5/2019 iron studies within normal
recommend lab repeat next 7days (no appointment needed. just come to
labs to have completed)
recommend increase daily water
refer to Endo (consult has been entered)
Thanks

––––––

To Dr. Lou—This is Grace, Jensen's caregiver. I am requesting an explanation
of the email you sent.
Specifically:
1-What are we to understand from:
testosterone 139 total(250–827 normal)
HH 11.1/33.1
2-What are we to understand from:
The anemia had increased since 5/2019 lab results of HH 12.8/37.8
6/28/2019FIt cards-negative and 5/2019 iron studies within normal
3-We do understand that we are to come for blood work. What labs will be
tested?
Thank you,
Grace (and Jensen)

––––––

(response from Dr. Lou)
the labs are to recheck your testosterone and LH hormones.
HH is your hemoglobin and hematocrit levels
FIT cards were the cards sent back with the stool samples that check for
hidden blood in the stool.
A visit to meet with me is NOT NEEDED.
thanks

––––––

Caregiver burden is the extent to which caregiving affects the emotional, social, financial, physical, and spiritual functioning of a caregiver (Zarit et al., 1986). We note that the term *burden* is not valenced necessarily as positive or negative, but rather is a measure of the expense of resources such as time, health, money, emotion, energy, etc. In Grace's email exchange from the patient portal, we can see that the provider and caregiver are speaking, literally, two different languages. The provider writes in medicalese and medical shorthand, and despite Viv's request for clarity and meaning, none is achieved. In fact, Grace and Jensen are told not to come and see the provider in person, and this was "shouted out to them" by writing in all caps that a visit "WAS NOT NEEDED." *Caregiver communication burden* is the summative force of perceived, experienced, and anticipated communication interaction for the caregiver with patient, providers, family, and system. Communication can exacerbate stress, depression, and anger; it calls on the most precious resource available to the caregiver: time (Wttenberg-Lyles et al., 2012).

The communication burden of caregivers, we believe, contributes mightily to the negative caregiver outcomes we have described in this chapter. Communication challenges include difficulty obtaining information and illness information overload, which impedes caregivers' ability to understand words and concepts (Chae et al., 2016), and confusion about complex instructions for the care and management of chronic disease (Wittenberg-Lyles et al., 2013). The use of complex medical jargon, an absence of physician–caregiver communication, and lack of medical preparation for care all contribute to communication challenges that cause caregiver distress (Given et al., 2011; Sterling, 2014) and caregiver burden.

When caregivers avoid communication about disease, it can contribute to caregiver depression (Geng et al., 2018), and caregivers who have difficulty accepting and talking about the illness experience complicated grief symptoms (Kramer et al., 2010). Caregivers desire training and preparation for their labors, and almost all caregivers report needing more help and information with a variety of topics related to caregiving. The greatest concerns to caregivers involves keeping their care recipient safe, managing their own stress, and making care decisions, especially as they impact end-of-life care (National Alliance for Caregiving and United Healthcare, 2011).

THE COMMUNICATION–HEALTH LITERACY CONNECTION

The interactional processes of health communication is a communicative and interactive component of health literacy, with health literacy being the end goal of health communication. (Heath, 2017; Ishikawa & Kiuchi, 2010). Prior research has illustrated that both concepts are relevant to the caregiving role, with demonstrated improvement following individualized caregiver education (Cianfrocca et al., 2018; Dingley et al., 2017). The caregiver's ability to find information and ask for help is a key factor in obtaining supportive resources for caregiving tasks and having additional resources lowers caregiver stress (Empeno et al., 2011). Improving the caregiver's ability to talk about chronic disease mediates coping and positively impacts stress (Fletcher et al., 2012). The ability and willingness to share information about chronic illness improves patient quality of life (Lai et al., 2016) and enhances the relational quality between patient and caregiver, which lowers caregiver depressive symptoms (Hou et al., 2018).

Information needs are high, and caregiver use of and reception to technology underscores this need. Regardless of age, caregivers outpace non-caregivers in the acquisition and use of e-information, especially information that helps in the delivery, understanding, coordination, and monitoring of care (Heynsbergh et al., 2018). Critical to learning more about the health information seeking needs of caregivers is understanding the places they turn to for trusted information. A quarter of caregivers have consulted information about medications, provider reviews, and hospital/care setting reviews. Family and friends remain a trusted source of information about care and support, with nearly 80% of caregivers relying on these avenues, compared to about 50% of non-caregivers (Schulz et al., 2018).

The proliferation of online access provides caregivers with countless online, asynchronous and synchronous support groups. Caregivers are able to benefit from their involvement in these forums that allow them to share their emotional toll, vent, locate the silver lining in their experience, seek advice from uniquely credible confidants, discuss the challenges of home, and adapt to the role of care-giver (Deifenbeck et al., 2017). Caregivers benefit from reflective discussions with healthcare professionals about the unique concerns of their caregiving situation, which does impact their sense of support and connectedness and increases their feeling of being prepared to deal with the day to day challenges with their care recipient (Slater et al., 2019).

Caregiver communication challenges reveal health literacy needs and con-tribute to caregiver distress/burden. Caregivers face communication difficulties related to caregiving tasks and decision-making. The use of complex medical jargon, an absence of physician–caregiver communication, and lack of education all contribute to communication challenges that cause caregiver distress (Given et al., 2011; Sterling, 2014). When caregivers avoid communication, it can con-tribute to caregiver depression (Geng et al., 2018) and caregivers who have diffi-culty accepting and talking about illness experience complicated grief symptoms (Kramer et al., 2010).

Of significance, we know that caregiver health literacy needs also impact patient outcomes. Unmet information needs about illness, treatment, and care-related in-formation are associated with increased patient physical symptoms, anxiety, and lower quality of life (Wang et al., 2018). Adverse effects of caregiver health literacy barriers on patient outcomes include misunderstanding prescription medication directions, inadequate knowledge of cancer and treatment effects (US Department of Health and Human Services, 2018), inability to assist with safe and effective home medication use (Roter et al., 2017), and risk of hospital readmission for the patient (Rodakowski et al., 2017). Moreover, poor caregiver mental and physical health impacts the ability to communicate productively with clinical staff (Litzelman et al., 2016). Ineffective communication between clinicians and caregivers impedes caregiver learning (Lau et al., 2010) and can result in poor adherence that leaves patient pain undertreated (Mayahara, 2011; Miaskowski et al., 2001).

We believe that caregiver effectiveness and well-being can be improved through better communication and improved health literacy, which also improves patient outcomes. Family caregiver "mastery," defined as "the feeling of being in control of the care situation," is predictive of patient survival (Boele et al., 2017, p. 832). But more important than the feeling of control is the ability to achieve care for the recipient. The caregiver's ability to find information and ask for help is a key factor in obtaining supportive resources for caregiving tasks (Ferrell & Wittenberg, 2017; Northouse et al., 2010) and having additional resources lowers caregiver stress (Empeno et al., 2011). Improving the caregiver's ability to talk about the illness mediates coping and positively impacts the stress process (Fletcher et al., 2012). The ability and willingness to share information improves patient quality of life (Lai et al., 2016) and enhances relational quality between patient and caregiver, which lowers caregiver depressive symptoms (Hou et al., 2018). Educational sessions for caregivers improve caregiver quality of life (Borneman et al., 2015) and dyadic patient–caregiver educational interventions that include communication improve caregiver quality of life, emotional support, communication, and relational intimacy (Ferrell & Wittenberg, 2017). A greater understanding of the impact of caregiver health communication and health literacy will assist healthcare providers with identifying caregiver-specific (or caregiver centered) support, resources, and interventions that can foster improved health outcomes for patients with cancer or chronic illness (Yuen et al., 2018).

Although research has reported evidence that links an individual's health literacy to their own poor health outcomes (Berkman et al., 2011; Hersh et al., 2015; Wu et al., 2016), there is an increasing need to obtain a better understanding regarding the complex role of caregiving and how it is heavily predicated upon health literacy skills. When caregivers have knowledge about a health condition and understand how it affects the person with chronic illness, they have some degree of acceptance of the condition as a part of family life (Thompson et al., 2017). Consonant with a palliative care approach, family communication about the illness is better for the caregiver if the illness is acknowledged (Arestedt et al., 2014).

PALLIATIVE CARE IMPERATIVE FOR CHRONIC ILLNESS CARE

Common elements in most definitions of chronic illness include a multifaceted approach to care, over an extended period of time, and involve coordinated input from a wide range of healthcare providers. Of significance is the very rarely recognized role of family in supporting the management of chronic disease. The model of patient-centered care does not, at this time, include the family in equal partnership with the patient and provider (Whitehead et al., 2017), even though the majority of chronic disease management takes place at home, with caregivers having an immense and proven impact upon patient outcomes.

A key factor in the lack of attention to family caregivers in chronic illness is the failure of the healthcare system and providers to engage in direct discussions about treatment and quality of life, opting to discuss only routine maintenance of care exclusive of patient/family preferences and goals throughout the care trajectory. This approach limits an open awareness of chronic illness that does not support resource utilization nor include care for the family caregiver. We believe that a palliative care approach, through the involvement of palliative care providers or in trained healthcare providers that can engage in palliative care communication, will facilitate incorporation of the family caregiver and address their needs, thereby improving care to the family caregiver and subsequently positively impacting patient care.

Palliative care aims to relieve suffering and improve quality of life for both patients with serious, chronic, or terminal illness and their families. It is provided simultaneously with all other appropriate (curative or noncurative) treatments and thus is for all patients suffering from stressful, painful, debilitating symptoms. Palliative care is delivered by an interdisciplinary team comprised of physician, nurses, social workers, and chaplains and can include a range of other healthcare providers such as psychologists and pharmacists (Get Palliative Care, 2019). A hallmark feature of palliative care is that care recipient and family constitute the unit of care as they suffer in constellation with one another. The approach includes addressing the physical, psychological, social, and spiritual components of care.

Palliative care improves outcomes for both patients and family caregivers. Effectiveness reviews demonstrate that palliative care can improve patient and family satisfaction and experience of care; reduce days in the hospital; reduce 30-day re-admissions; and, especially toward the end-of-life, reduce total spending (Center to Advance Palliative Care, 2018). In oncology, palliative care improves quality of life and survival (Bakitas et al., 2017; Temel et al., 2010) and reduces symptom burden, financial burden, and emergency department visits for symptom management (Hallman & Newton, 2019). Family caregivers involved in palliative care have fewer unmet needs and reduced distress, feel more prepared for caregiving, and report improved vitality and social functioning (El-Jawahri et al., 2016).

Chronic illness demands more attention to palliative care communication as it attends to both the patient and family and serves to coordinate many factions across multiple care settings. Patient/family–provider communication is critical to a palliative care approach. Palliative care communication involves engaging in responsive communication about diagnosis, discussing factors influencing treatment decision-making, relaying and mediating communication among family members, and providing psychosocial counseling about difficult topics. Palliative care conversations are contextual, dependent upon the type of healthcare system, size and nature of the palliative care program available, clinical setting, and the availability of resources (Hui et al., 2018). As chronic illness involves many moving parts, palliative care discussions help with continuity across care settings and in transition management.

Palliative care improves communication with families by (a) clarifying goals of care with patients and families; (b) helping families select treatment and care settings that meet their goals; and (c) assisting with decisions to leave the hospital or withhold or withdraw death-prolonging treatment that does not align with the patient's end-of-life goals. This also includes discussing a range of topics;

encouraging the sharing of feelings and fears about the illness, treatment, and prognosis; and helping patients and family members find a sense of control and a search for meaning and life purpose (Ragan et al., 2008). Palliative care discussions facilitate the support, comfort, relief, and continuity possible as family is considered part of the unit of care. We will further unpack these discussions in Chapter 3.

A NARRATIVE LENS TO FAMILY CAREGIVING

Eminent medical anthropologist and Harvard psychiatrist, Arthur Kleinman, has also informed our understanding of the significance of the patient's experience and story. After decades of diagnosing and treating patients from numerous cultures, Kleinman notes that modern medical training neglects teaching clinicians to value the lived experience of the patient: he posits that intently listening to patients and families and their stories can teach healthcare providers to learn to respond compassionately to patients whose experiences are foreign to their own (Kleinman, 1988). Kleinman proposes eight questions to enhance communication and better assess the feelings, beliefs, and experiences of individuals regarding illness. These questions assist in understanding the person's explanatory model that can provide valuable insight into what is believed, what patients feel will help, and what is most important to the individual (Kleinman, 1988). Asking these eight questions and incorporating patients' answers into their treatment plans can help reduce the distance between witness (healthcare provider) and sufferer (patient/family). Kleinman most recently has produced a volume that honors the story of his and his late wife's experience with early onset dementia (Kleinman, 2019).

Narrative assumes that all forms of human communication can be seen fundamentally as stories, as interpretations of aspects of the world occurring in time and shaped by history, culture, and character (Fisher, 1987). Illness, like narrative, occurs within context at the same time it reshapes context, within relationships at the same time it reshapes them, and within a person's life at the same time that it reshapes that life. Caregivers engage in storytelling as a way of interpreting the illness journey. **Family illness narratives** are those stories that situate the informal caregiver's experiences and interpretations of a care recipient's illness. These narratives are a communicative attempt to make sense of disconnected fragments of experiences, loss, hope, shifting identity, change, and hope. Family dynamics are often included in these interpretive descriptions, as well as the challenges of providers, systems, and the patient herself or himself. As an illness journey shifts to the need for end-of-life care, patients and family members create stories to make sense of their healthcare experiences and process this shift. Similarly, the absence of communication about illness can lead to narratives that disorder human experiences and result in illness journeys that do not focus on pain management and quality of life.

Family illness narratives illumine an understanding of the illness for providers and caregivers (Sharf & Vanderford, 2003). These narratives incorporate the humanistic perspective of disease and illness as they extend beyond biological suffering and include the family experience with illness as related to changing roles, relationships, identities, and the intense labors of caregiving (Sharf & Vanderford, 2003). The inclusion of family illness narratives in research and care innovations is an approach that challenges the assumptions of existing knowledge, thus enabling us to highlight and focus on the communicative domain of chronic illness. Throughout this volume we share the stories, words, and experiences of caregivers through their family narratives in the context of chronic illness. These families reveal their struggles to oppose, control, manage, avoid, and partner with the medical world and its communications as well as pre-existing family communication patterns.

FAMILY CAREGIVER COMMUNICATION TYPES

When a family member is diagnosed with a chronic illness, family communication patterns are highlighted by the illness crisis. Family communication patterns develop from implicit and explicit rules for communicating within a family system. Family rules govern appropriate topics and frequency of discussion (family **conversation**) and a hierarchy among family members (family **conformity**). Patterns of family conversation and family conformity range from high to low to form specific communication behaviors among family members and define the communication environment for that group of people (Fitzpatrick, 2004). Based on varying communication patterns, this volume presents the Family Caregiver Communication Typology, which defines four caregiver types: Manager, Carrier, Partner, and Lone caregivers.

The motives of the caregiver are shaped significantly by and are a product of family communication patterns. The conversation and conformity patterns that have surrounded the caregiver have always had a significant impact on the communication and behaviors they enact—long before illness and caregiving began. But in the face of chronic illness, each caregiver is coping as they navigate sometimes very long caregiving tenures. No matter the coping style, the labors and sacrifices they offer are significant actions that contribute to patient care that would not be possible otherwise. It's worth underscoring that caregiving is not always met with selflessness and willingness. The cost of caregiving, as we have detailed in this volume, is life altering.

We first began developing the typology of caregivers in 2010. It quickly became clear in presentations and talks about the types that some were perceived as more favorable for audiences (made up primarily of clinical nurses) or perceived as being more functional and successful. But as we have learned more and more about the typology, we want to emphasize that each caregiver type has strengths and weaknesses, and each caregiver type arrives at good patient and caregiver outcomes **differently**. So, yes, there are barriers for each type in arriving at the best care for the caregiver and the care recipient, as well as pathways for each that need fortification and support. The communication patterns experienced and engaged by each type set the stage for the caregiver communication burden experienced and the resources that a caregiver will be able to locate and access.

The Family Caregiver Communication Typology illustrates how family caregivers communicate differently and have different communication, information and support needs. Caregivers may need differing support depending on the care recipient's condition, as well as their own strengths, health literacy skills, available resources, and nonmedical determinates. An often-heard phrase in the health literacy field is "You can't tell by looking." This is used to dispel the common misconception often shared by healthcare providers that they can tell who has low health literacy by how a person looks, speaks, or even by their occupation. We suggest adding another "myth breaker" by proffering: "You can't tell by looking who may be struggling with their caregiver role."

Communication with families can be challenging for healthcare providers because family members may avoid communication about the illness, certain family members can be excluded from decision-making, and there is a propensity for the patient and family to hide their feelings from one another (Caughlin et al., 2011; Friedemann & Buckwalter, 2014). Different communication styles among family members contribute to communication difficulties and a family member's illness can trigger the re-emergence of previous family conflicts (Demiris et al., 2012). When providers know about the communities they serve, their beliefs and perceptions, and the existing resources, they can further support caregiver engagement. Engaging caregivers as part of the care team and assessing risk stratification screening and strategies to optimize caregiver well-being may enhance patient-reported outcomes and quality of care (Litzelman et al., 2016).

OUR APPROACH TO FAMILY CAREGIVING AND THE DATA

Our approach to understanding more about family caregiving is influenced by previous work about the family and its dynamics. An important element in this process of understanding is defining the concept of *family*. Baxter and Braithwaite's description serves as a starting place for this definition, which includes familial relationships over time designated by commitment, relations created through biology/law/affection, kinship organization, ongoing interdependence, and institutionalization (Floyd et al., 2006). But there are gaps in this conceptualization that we fill here with our efforts to know more about the family caregiver. Specifically, we employ *role* as our conceptual lens to identify family. A role lens considers the emotional attachment and patterns of interaction defined by the way people act and interact (Floyd et al., 2006). This notion of family is thus constituted by *communication*.

Adding to this communication definition of family, we also include a recent LGBTQ+ definitional study that conceptualizes family as *unconditional* in terms of love, support, and acceptance (Willes et al., 2019). Embracing our beliefs that participants (caregivers, care recipients) are the authentic source of knowledge that informs the work in this volume, we share our working definition of family here: family includes the people the participant identifies as family (Goldsmith et al., 2015; Wittenberg et al., 2019). The family, as a unit, is central to the caregiving enterprise, as the function and structure of a family informs the readiness for care, the navigation of conflict, and the magnification and amelioration of the care recipient's/caregiver's internal struggle with illness (Anderson & White, 2018). Although our approach and conceptualization of family is present in academic and everyday life circles, most healthcare stakeholders continue to acknowledge only the legal recognition of family. This is one example of how reality outpaces policy in healthcare.

Caregiver communication research has neglected to account for the influence of time and communication patterns on how family members interact. The illness experiences collected for this volume cover high- and low-intensity caregiving over short and longer periods of time. Family illness narratives were collected using ethnomethods ranging from observation to interview to self-reported narratives. Over the last 10 years, we have been programmatic in our efforts to study the family caregiver across care settings, illnesses, and in varying geographic locations. To organize caregivers by type, they all were given the Family Caregiver Communication Tool (see Chapter 4 of this volume) to determine if they were a Manager, Partner, Carrier, or Lone caregiver. Privileging the caregiver's voice was a priority in every effort to learn about this underserved stakeholder. As family relationships are exposed to change—sometimes drastic and sometimes incremental—we believe the experiences are manifested in family dialogue with each other and with healthcare providers and systems. Studying the family system and the story of the family educates providers about the communication burden present for the family caregiver (Kirby et al., 2018).

OUR FEATURED CAREGIVERS

Maggie Burkhart

Maggie has been a grant coordinator for a large school system in the south and for the last five years has worked as a grant specialist for a large research university in the same region. She is a strong communicator and is a skilled at networking people with solutions. She is the fourth of four kids and now in her late 50s has her own family with two grown children and a 30-year marriage. Her own dad was an alcoholic, and she recognizes the impact that experience has had on her as an adult—needing to find ways to control the uncontrollable around her. Growing up, her household was economically depressed, and her success in work has always been a stabilizing force in her adult life.

Maggie is a completer in all aspects of life. She earned a bachelor's and master's degree in close succession, paying her own way throughout. She enjoys arriving at the conclusion of tasks and is eager to fill the needs of those around her. In addition to her own professional successes, she married an ordained clergy who has served in high-level administrative positions in the church and seminaries, requiring Maggie's involvement and personal skill set of networking and ensuring projects are moved forward and finished.

Maggie is the youngest among her siblings. She describes their order of birth as fairly typical in impacting their role and identity. As the youngest, she was somewhat freer than the rest in cutting her own path and feeling less dependent on the approval of her parents in making life decisions. She had been self-reliant all along, and this has come as a source of comfort and structure for her.

Sharon Jenks

For the last two decades Sharon has worked closely with two law partners and served as their office manager. She has seen the practice grow from carrying a yearly deficit to a healthy and wealthy firm committed to close client attention and success. Her close connection and loyalty with the practice had given her tremendous financial stability and independence. After having a family with three children, now grown, Sharon left her marriage. Once on her own, she met and married Kelley, and together they became a new family, with kids on both sides, and new grandchildren arriving in rapid succession. The work of blending their family elements together came at a fairly high cost of energy and time for Sharon. Outstanding hurt and loss existed for two of the children, and Sharon's new wife had a mother who was not welcoming.

In any case, the work of the family seemed to fill Sharon's time and energy, and the burdens of her previous marriage were gone, but her new spouse and extended family included its own new labors and costs. Sharon would often leave her own needs until last, putting resources and effort toward the children and grandchildren. She found support and solace in her work but also in a long-time counselor she had been seeing for nearly a decade. This counselor had shepherded her through the trying times of her divorce and the challenges of integrating her family.

Over time, Sharon had attended less and less to her own health. Her weight had crept up on her, and she sought excuses to miss her own yearly physical. Although her partner was into fitness and exercise, Sharon never could find time to prioritize this in her busy work and family schedule.

Estella Rodriguez

Estella lived about three hours from the other parts of her family and raised her four children with her spouse in South Texas. Her family had immigrated from Chiapas, Mexico, to the United States two years before she was born; Estella and her three siblings grew up in a diverse South Texas community that represented first- and second-generation Americans with strong ties and family in Mexico.

Estella's dad carved out stable employment as a brick layer when she was a little girl, but over time he took on larger administrative responsibilities for building projects that included housing developments and even corporate building sites, and by his early 40s he was mostly performing site visits and monitoring construction budgets. The family celebrated as Estella's parents were able to comfortably retire to a lovely rural community and enjoy life with less work. Meanwhile, their now-adult children worked tirelessly in their own career paths as they now each had spouses and families to support. Estella had taken the path of accountancy and worked as a payroll officer for regional Environmental Protection Agency offices in Texas. Her employment was very steady, and she had advanced in her career in the midst of being a parent of four boys under the age of 10. Her sister lived close by, and two brothers were about two hours away. Each sibling had a rigorous work ethic and wanted to reflect the values and commitments their parents had demonstrated to them.

Viv Gray

Planning to be an artist, Viv attended college to train for that creative career path. She grew up in central Nebraska in a family of academic parents and two other siblings, also with academic prowess. Viv's interests, goals, and endeavors were out of character for her family system. She was creative, nonlinear, and open to the journey along the way. With parents and siblings less than interested in the path less traveled that was calling her, Viv was never in close contact with the family. And, in fact, her other two siblings seemed to harbor their own disconnected feelings from their parents, and it was rare that they would all get together or stay in regular touch. Viv traveled abroad on her own for three years, intermittently teaching English and exploring new and unknown places. After a lot of life experience and adventure, she returned to the United States with the intention of opening her own pottery studio and gallery.

As the years passed, differences within her nuclear family were fortified by life choices, geographical placement, and unprocessed/unspoken conflict. Viv embraced her own solitary path and carved out new pseudo-family structures along the way, which lasted for a time and then faded away. By her 40s, she was still single with no children, and her artistic aspirations had not proven successful. Although continuing her own pottery business on the side, Viv was a vet technician and worked part time. She rarely saw her family, and the modern technologies of email and text were not a method of connection they embraced. At the age of 43, without warning, a childhood friend reappeared in her life via another shared friend, and Viv suddenly found herself in a loving and sustained partnership for the first time.

OVERVIEW OF THE BOOK

We who write about illness, caregiving, death, and dying are particularly attuned to the stories of illness from friends and loved ones. These get shared in desperation, in gratitude, and also in those moments in which both the sufferer of chronic illness and her family caregiver are enmeshed in the dilemma of figuring out what to do next. These stories point up two verities: a really sick person is at the mercy of his caregiver(s), and the way of practicing medicine in the United States adds to the inherent misery of being ill by obfuscating information about the illness and how best to treat it. Telling an illness story, particularly to healthcare providers, reifies for patients and caregivers that their experience is unique—that its hearing may compel providers to treat the person, not the disease. The stories of our caregivers will carry into Chapter 2 where caregiver health literacy and burden will reveal caregiving communication challenges related to health literacy barriers. Chapter 3 highlights palliative care as an approach for helping family caregivers to understand disease and treatment. Three illness journeys are described (isolated, rescued, comforted) to further detail how communication and health literacy impact the caregiver and patient. The Family Caregiver Communication Typology we will share in Chapter 4 illustrates the variance among family caregivers in terms of communication and health literacy. In Chapters 5 to 8, we detail each of the four caregiver types by sharing the features and patterns of each caregiver type. We tell the story of these four types of caregivers and articulate their communication patterns and how those patterns impact caregiving. Between the caregiver type chapters, we intersperse four spotlights written to focus, direct, and illuminate caregiver narratives and reflections about the most formidable and invisible costs of caregiving. While effective communication and person-centered care are essential for all caregivers and care recipients, we end the volume with Chapter 9 suggesting that effective healthcare provider communication and health literacy interventions can be further tailored to meet the unique characteristics, needs, and preferences of each of the four caregiver types.

REFERENCES

Aldridge, M. D., & Bradley, E. H. (2017). Epidemiology and patterns of care at the end of life: Rising complexity, shifts in care patterns and sites of death. *Health Affairs (Millwood), 36*(7), 1175–1183. https://doi.org/10.1377/hlthaff.2017.0182

Alzheimer's Association. (2016). 2016 Alzheimer's disease facts and figures. *Alzheimer's Dementia: Journal of Alzheimer's Association, 12*(4), 459–509.

Anderson, E., & White, K. (2018). "This is what family does": The family experience of caring for serious illness. *American Journal of Hospice and Palliative Medicine, 35*(2), 348–354. https://doi.org/10.1177/1049909117709251

Arestedt, L., Persson, C., & Benzein, E. (2014). Living as a family in the midst of chronic illness. *Scandinavian Journal of Caring Science, 28*(1), 29–37. https://doi.org/10.1111/scs.12023

Ascher, E. A., Sturm, V. E., Seider, B. H., Holley, S. R., Miller, B. L., & Levenson, R. W. (2010). Relationship satisfaction and emotional language in frontotemporal dementia and Alzheimer disease patients and spousal caregivers. *Alzheimer Disease Association Disorders, 24*(1), 49–55.

Ashida, S., Marcum, C. S., & Koehly, L. M. (2017). Unmet expectations in Alzheimer's family caregiving: Interactional characteristics associated with perceived under-contribution. *Gerontologist, 58*(2), e46–e55. https://doi.org/10.1093.geront/gnx141

Bakitas, M. A., El-Jawahri, A., Farquhar, M., Ferrell, B., Grudzen, C., Higginson, I., . . . Smith, T. J. (2017). The TEAM approach to improving oncology outcomes by incorporating palliative care in practice. *Journal of Oncology Practice, 13*(9), 557–566. https://doi.org/10.1200/JOP.2017.022939

Bangerter, L., Griffin, J., & Dunlay, S. (2018). Qualitative study of challenges of caring for a person with heart failure. *Geriatric Nursing, 39*(4), 443–449.

Berkman, N., Sheridan, S., Donahue, K., Halpern, D., Viera, A., Crotty, K., & Viswanathan, M. (2011). *Health literacy interventions and outcomes: An updated systematic review* (Evidence report/technology assessment no. 199). Rockville, MD: Agency for Healthcare Research and Quality.

Berry, L., Dulwadi, S. M., & Jacobson, J. (2017). What family caregivers need to care for a loved one with cancer. *Journal of Oncology Practitioners, 13*(1), 35–41. https://doi.org/10.1200/JOP.2016.017913

Boele, F. W., Given, C. W., Given, B. A., Donovan, H. S., Schulz, R., Weimer, J. M., . . . Sherwood, P. R. (2017). Family caregivers' level of mastery predicts survival of patients with glioblastoma: A preliminary report. *Cancer, 123*(5), 832–840. https://doi.org/10.1002/cncr.30428

Borneman, T., Sun, V., Williams, A. C., Fujinami, R., Del Ferraro, C., Burhenn, P. S., . . . Buga, S. (2015). Support for patients and family caregivers in lung cancer: Educational components of an interdisciplinary palliative care intervention. *Journal of Hospice & Palliative Nursing, 17*(4), 309–318. https://doi.org/10.1097/NJH.0000000000000165

Brody, J. (2016). Supporting children who serve as caregivers. *New York Times.*

Cagle, J., Bunting, M., Kelemen, A., Lee, J., Terry, D., & Harris, R. (2017). Psychosocial needs and interventions for heart failure patients and families receiving palliative care support: A systematic review. *Heart Failure Review, 22*, 565–580. https://doi.org/10.1007/s10741-017-9596-5

Cagle, J., & Munn, J. (2012). Long distance caregiving: A systematic review of the literature. *Journal of Gerontological Social Work, 55*(8), 682–707. https://doi.org/10.1080/01634372.2012.703763

Caughlin, J. P., Mikucki-Enyart, S., Middelton, A., Stone, A., & Brown, L. (2011). Being open without talking about it: A rhetorical/normative approach to understanding topic avoidance in families after a lung cancer diagnosis. *Communication Monographs, 78*(4), 409–436. https://doi.org/10.1080/03637751.2011.618141

Center to Advance Palliative Care. (2018, February 28). *Palliative care continues its annual growth trend.* Retrieved from https://www.capc.org/about/press-media/press-releases/2018-2-28/palliative-care-continues-its-annual-growth-trend-according-latest-center-advance-palliative-care-analysis/

Centers for Disease Control. (2019). *Heart disease facts.* Retrieved from https://www.cdc.gov/heartdisease/facts.htm

Chae, J., Lee, C. J., & Jensen, J. D. (2016). Correlates of cancer information overload: Focusing on individual ability and motivation. *Health Communication, 31*(5), 626–634. https://doi.org/10.1080/10410236.2014.986026

Cianfrocca, C., Caponnetto, V., Donati, D., Lancia, L., Tartaglini, D., & Di Stasio, E. (2018). The effects of a multidisciplinary education course on the burden, health literacy and needs of family caregivers. *Applied Nursing Research, 44,* 100–106. https://doi.org/10.1016/j.apnr.2018.10.004

Coller, R., & Kuo, A. (2016). Social determinants of child health. In A. Kuo, R. Koller, S. S. Brown, & M. Blair (Eds.), *Child health: A population perspective* (pp. 79–110). New York, NY: Oxford University Press.

Costa, M., & Pereira, M. (2017). Predictors and moderators of quality of life in caregivers of amputee patients by type 2 diabetes. *Scandinavian Journal of Caring Science, 32*(2), 933–942. https://doi.org/10.1111/scs.12528

Damjanovic, A., Yang, Y., Glaser, R., Kiecolt-Glaser, J., Nguyen, H., Laskowski, B., . . . Weng, N. P. (2007). Accelerated telomere erosion is associated with a declining immune function of caregivers of Alzheimer's disease patients. *Journal of Immunology, 179*(6), 4249–4254.

Dassel, K. B., Carr, D. C., & Vitaliano, P. (2015). Does caring for a spouse with dementia accelerate cognitive decline? Findings from the health and retirement study. *Gerontologist, 57*(2), 319–328.

Deifenbeck, C., Klemm, P., & Hayes, E. (2017). Anonymous meltdown: Content themes emerging in a nonfacilitated, peer-only, unstructured, anonymous online support group for family caregivers. *Computers, Informatics, Nursing, 35*(12), 630–638. https://doi.org/10.1097/CIN.0000000000000376

Demiris, G., Parker Oliver, D., Wittenberg-Lyles, E., Washington, K., Doorenbos, A., Rue, T., & Berry, D. (2012). A noninferiority trial of a problem-solving intervention for hospice caregivers: In person versus videophone. *Journal of Palliative Medicine, 15*(6), 653–660. https://doi.org/10.1089/jpm.2011.0488

Demitz, C. (2017). Caregiving and its impact on women. *Michigan State University Extension.* Retrieved from https://www.canr.msu.edu/news/caregiving_and_its_impact_on_women

Dingley, C. E., Clayton, M., Lai, D., Doyon, K., Reblin, M., & Ellington, L. (2017). Caregiver activation and home hospice nurse communication in advanced cancer care. *Cancer Nursing, 40*(5), E38–E50. https://doi.org/10.1097/NCC.0000000000000429

El-Jawahri, A., LeBlanc, T., VanDusen, H., Traeger, L., Greer, J. A., Pirl, W. F., . . . Temel, J. S. (2016). Effect of inpatient palliative care on quality of life 2 weeks after hematopoietic stem cell transplantation: A randomized clinical trial. *JAMA, 316*(20), 2094–2103. https://doi.org/10.1001/jama.2016.16786

Empeno, J., Raming, N. T., Irwin, S. A., Nelesen, R. A., & Lloyd, L. S. (2011). The hospice caregiver support project: Providing support to reduce caregiver stress. *Journal of Palliative Medicine, 14*(5), 593–597. https://doi.org/10.1089/jpm.2010.0520

Espinoza, R. (2014). *Out and visible: The experiences and attitudes of lesbian, gay, bisexual and transgender older adults, ages 45–75.* New York, NY: SAGE.

Family Caregiver Alliance. (2006). *Caregiver health.* Retrieved from https://www.caregiver.org/caregiver-health

Family Caregiver Alliance. (2017). *Selected long-term care statistics.* Retrieved from https://www.caregiver.org/selected-long-term-care-statistics

Family Caregiver Alliance. (2019). *Women and caregiving.* Retrieved from https://www.caregiver.org/women-and-caregiving-facts-and-figures

Ferrell, B., & Wittenberg, E. (2017). A review of family caregiving intervention trials in oncology. *Cancer, 67*(4), 318–325. https://doi.org/10.3322/caac.21396

Fisher, W. (1987). *Human communication as narration: Toward a philosophy of reason, value, and action.* Columbia: University of South Carolina Press.

Fitzpatrick, M. A. (2004). Family communication patterns theory: Observations on its development and application. *Journal of Family Communication, 4*(3–4), 167–179.

Fletcher, B. S., Miaskowski, C., Given, B., & Schumacher, K. (2012). The cancer family caregiving experience: An updated and expanded conceptual model. *European Journal of Oncology Nursing, 16*(4), 387–398. https://doi.org/10.1016/j.ejon.2011.09.001

Floyd, K., Mikkelson, A., & Judd, J. (2006). Defining the family through relationships. In L. Turner & R. West (Eds.), *The family communication sourcebook* (pp. 21–42). Thousand Oaks, CA: SAGE.

Friedemann, M.-L., & Buckwalter, K. C. (2014). Family caregiver role and burden related to gender and family relationships. *Journal of Family Nursing, 20*(3), 313–336. https://doi.org/10.1177/1074840714532715

Friedman, A. L., Kachur, R. E., Noar, S. M., & McFarlane, M. (2016). Health communication and social marketing campaigns for sexually transmitted disease prevention and control: What Is the evidence of their effectiveness? *Sexually Transmitted Diseases, 43*(Suppl 2), S83–S101. https://doi.org/10.1097/olq.0000000000000286

Fujinami, R., Sun, V., Zachariah, F., Uman, G., Grant, M., & Ferrell, B. (2015). Family caregivers' distress levels related to quality of life, burden, and preparedness. *Psycho-Oncology, 24*(1), 54–62. https://doi.org/10.1002/pon.3562

Galarraga, M., & Llahan, S. (2018). Quality of life for carers of people with type 2 diabetes: A literature review. *Journal of Diabetes Nursing, 22*(1), 1–8.

Geng, H. M., Chuang, D. M., Yang, F., Yang, Y., Liu, W. M., Liu, L. H., & Tian, H. M. (2018). Prevalence and determinants of depression in caregivers of cancer patients: A systematic review and meta-analysis. *Medicine (Baltimore), 97*(39), e11863. https://doi.org/10.1097/MD.0000000000011863

Get Palliative Care. (2019). *What is palliative care?* Retrieved from https://getpalliativecare.org/whatis/

Given, B. A., Sherwood, P., & Given, C. W. (2011). Support for caregivers of cancer patients: Transition after active treatment. *Cancer Epidemiological Biomarkers Prevention, 20*(10), 2015–2021. https://doi.org/10.1158/1055-9965.EPI-11-0611

Goldsmith, J., Wittenberg, E., Small Platt, C., Innarino, N., & Reno, J. (2015). Family caregiver communication in oncology: Advancing a typology. *Psycho-Oncology, 25*(4), 463–470. https://doi.org/10.1002/PON.3862

Hallman, K., & Newton, S. (2019). Outpatient palliative care: A case study illustrating clinic support offered to patients receiving cancer treatment. *Clinical Journal of Oncology Nursing, 23*(2), 203–208. https://doi.org/10.1188/19.CJON.203-208

Heath, S. (2017, June 13). The difference between patient education and health literacy. *Patient Engagement.* Retrieved from https://patientengagementhit.com/news/the-difference-between-patient-education-and-health-literacy

Hersh, L., Salzman, B., & Snyderman, D. (2015). Health literacy in primary care practice. *American Family Physician, 92*(2), 118–124. https://www.ncbi.nlm.nih.gov/pubmed/26176370

Heynsbergh, N., Heckel, L., Botti, M., & Livingston, P. (2018). Feasibility, useability and acceptability of technology-based interventions for information cancer carers: A systematic review. *BMC Cancer, 18*, 244.

Hicks, K., Downey, L., Engelberg, R., Fausto, J., Starks, H., Dunlap, B., . . . Curtis, R. (2018). Predictors of death in the hospital for patients with chronic serious illness. *Journal of Palliative Medicine, 21*(3), 307–313. https://doi.org/10.1089/jpm.2017.0127

Hou, W. K., Lau, K. M., Shum, T. C. Y., Cheng, A. C. K., & Lee, T. M. C. (2018). Do concordances of social support and relationship quality predict psychological distress and well-being of cancer patients and caregivers? *European Journal of Cancer Care (Engl), 27*(4), e12857. https://doi.org/10.1111/ecc.12857

Hsieh, S., Irish, M., Daveson, N., Hodges, J. R., & Piquet, O. (2013). When one loses empathy; its effect on carers of patients with dementia. *Journal of Geriatric Psychiatry and Neurology, 26*(3), 174–184.

Hui, D., Hannon, B. L., Zimmermann, C., & Bruera, E. (2018). Improving patient and caregiver outcomes in oncology: Team-based, timely, and targeted palliative care. *Cancer, 68*(5), 356–376. https://doi.org/10.3322/caac.21490

Institute of Medicine. (2015). *Improving quality and honoring individual preferences near the end of life.* Washington, DC: National Academy Press.

Institute on Aging. (2019). *Women as caregivers.* Retrieved from https://www.ioaging.org/aging-in-america#caregivers

Ishikawa, H., & Kiuchi, T. (2010). Health literacy and health communication. *Biopsychosocial Medicine, 4*, 18. https://doi.org/10.1186/1751-0759-4-18

Kirby, E., Lwin, Z., Kenny, K., Broom, A., Birman, H., & Good, P. (2018). "It doesn't exist . . .": Negotiating palliative care from a culturally and linguistically diverse patient and caregiver perspective. *BMC Palliative Care, 17*(1), 90. https://doi.org/10.1186/s12904-018-0343-z

Kleinman, A. (1988). *The illness narratives: Suffering, healing, and the human condition.* New York, NY: Basic Books.

Kleinman, A. (2019). *The soul of care: The moral education of husband and doctor.* New York, NY: Viking.

Kramer, B. J., Kavanaugh, M., Trentham-Dietz, A., Walsh, M., & Yonker, J. A. (2010). Complicated grief symptoms in caregivers of persons with lung cancer: The role of family conflict, intrapsychic strains, and hospice utilization. *Omega (Westport), 62*(3), 201–220. https://doi.org/10.2190/om.62.3.a

Lai, C., Borrelli, B., Ciurluini, P., & Aceto, P. (2016). Sharing information about cancer with one's family is associated with improved quality of life. *Psycho-Oncology.* https://doi.org/10.1002/pon.4334

Lau, D. T., Berman, R., Halpern, L., Pickard, A. S., Schrauf, R., & Witt, W. (2010). Exploring factors that influence informal caregiving in medication management for home hospice patients. *Journal of Palliative Medicine, 13*(9), 1085–1090. https://doi.org/10.1089/jpm.2010.0082

Leontis, L., & Hess-Fischl, A. (2019). Type 2 diabetes facts and tips. *Endocrineweb.* Retrieved from https://www.endocrineweb.com/conditions/type-2-diabetes/type-2-diabetes-facts-tips

Litzelman, K., Kent, E. E., Mollica, M., & Rowland, J. H. (2016). How does caregiver well-being relate to perceived quality of care in patients with cancer? Exploring associations and pathways. *Journal of Clinical Oncology, 34*(29), 3554–3561. https://doi.org/10.1200/JCO.2016.67.3434

Martin, C., Shrestha, A., Burton, M., Collins, K., & Wyld, L. (2019). How are caregivers involved in treatment decision making for older people with dementia and a new diagnosis of cancer? *Psycho-Oncology, 28*(6), 1197–1206. https://doi.org/10.1002/pon.5070

Mayahara, M. (2011). Pain medication management by hospice caregivers. *Pain, 12*(4), 27. https://doi.org/10.1016/j.jpain.2011.02.111

Merrilees, J. (2016). The impact of dementia on family caregivers: What is research teaching us? *Current Neurological Neuroscience Reports, 16*(10), 88. https://doi.org/10.1007/s119100-016-0692-z

MetLife Mature Market Group. (2011, June). *The MetLife study of working caregivers and employer health costs: Double jeopardy for baby boomers caring for their parents.* Retrieved from https://www.caregiving.org/wp-content/uploads/2011/06/mmi-caregiving-costs-working-caregivers.pdf

Miaskowski, C., Dodd, M. J., West, C., Paul, S. M., Tripathy, D., Koo, P., & Schumacher, K. (2001). Lack of adherence with the analgesic regimen: A significant barrier to effective cancer pain management. *Journal of Clinical Oncology, 19*(23), 4275–4279. https://doi.org/10.1200/JCO.2001.19.23.4275

Milliken, A., Mahoney, E., Mahoney, K., Mignosa, K., Rodriguez, I., Cuchetti, C., & Inoue, M. (2019). "I'm just trying to cope for both of us": Challenges and supports of family caregivers in participant-directed programs. *Journal of Gerontological Social Work, 62*(2), 149–171. https://doi.org/10.1080/01634372.2018.1475438

Moss, K., Kurzawa, C., Daly, B., & Prince-Paul, M. (2019). Identifying and addressing family caregiver anxiety. *Journal of Hospice and Palliative Nursing, 21*(1), 14–20. https://doi.org/10.1097/NJH.0000000000000489

National Alliance for Caregiving. (2018, January). *From insight to advocacy: Addressing family caregiving as a national public health issue.* Retrieved from http://www.caregiving.org/wp-content/uploads/2018/01/From-Insight-to-Advocacy_2017_FINAL.pdf

National Alliance for Caregiving and AARP. (2015). *Caregiving in the US.* Retrieved from https://www.caregiving.org/research/caregivingusa/

National Alliance for Caregiving and United Healthcare. (2011). *e-Connected family caregiver: Bringing caregiving into the 21st century.* Retrieved from https://www.caregiving.org/data/FINAL_eConnected_Family_Caregiver_Study_Jan%202011.pdf

Nipp, R., El-Jawahri, A., Fishbein, J., Gallagher, E. R., Stagl, J. M., Park, E. R., . . . Temel, J. S. (2016). Factors associated with depression and anxiety symptoms in family caregivers of patients with incurable cancer. *Annals of Oncology, 27*(8), 1607–1612.

Northouse, L. L., Katapodi, M. C., Song, L., Zhang, L., & Mood, D. W. (2010). Interventions with family caregivers of cancer patients: Meta-analysis of randomized trials. *Cancer, 60*(5), 317–339. https://doi.org/10.3322/caac.20081

O'Dwyer, S., Moyle, W., Zimmer-Gembeck, M., & De Leo, D. (2016). Suicidal ideation in family carers of people with dementia. *Aging Mental Health, 20*(2), 222–230.

Office of Disease Prevention and Health Promotion. (2019). *Overview of health communication and health literacy.* Retrieved from https://health.gov/communication/about.asp

Parnell, T. A. (2015). *Health literacy in nursing: Providing person-centered care.* New York, NY: Springer.

Pressler, S., Gradus-Pizlo, I., Chubinski, S., Smith, G., Wheeler, S., Sloan, R., & Jung, M. (2013). Family careivers of patients with heart failure: A longitudinal study. *Journal of Cardiovascular Nursing, 28*(5), 417–428.

Ragan, S., Wittenberg-Lyles, E., Goldsmith, J., & Sanchez-Reilly, S. (2008). *Communication as comfort: Multiple voices in palliative care.* New York, NY: Routledge, Taylor and Francis.

Ramchand, R., Tanielian, T., Fisher, M., Vaughan, C., Trail, T., Batka, C., . . . Ghosh-Dastidar, B. (2014). Key facts and statistics from the Rand Military Caregivers Study. *Rand Corporation.* Retrieved from https://www.rand.org/pubs/presentations/PT124.html

Ream, E., VH, P., Oakley, C., Richardson, A., Taylor, C., & Verity, R. (2013). Informal carers' experiences and needs when supporting patients through chemotherapy: A mixed method study. *European Journal of Cancer Care (Engl), 22*(6), 797–806. https://doi.org/10.1111/ecc.12083

Reigada, C., Pais-Ribeiro, J., Novellas, A., & Gonçalves, E. (2015). The caregiver role in palliative care: A systematic review of the literature. *Health Care Current Reviews, 3*(2), 143. https://doi.org/10.4172/2375-4273.1000143

Reinhard, S., Feinberg, L., Choula, R., & Houser, A. (2015). Valuing the invaluable: 2015 update. *AARP Public Policy Institute.* Retrieved from https://www.aarp.org/content/dam/aarp/ppi/2015/valuing-the-invaluable-2015-update-new.pdf

Reinhard, S., Young, H., Levine, C., Kelly, K., Choula, R., & Accius, J. (2019). Home alone revisited: Family caregivers providing complex care. *AARP.* Retrieved from https://www.aarp.org/ppi/info-2018/home-alone-family-caregivers-providing-complex-chronic-care.html

Rodakowski, J., Rocco, P. B., Ortiz, M., Folb, B., Schulz, R., Morton, S. C., . . . James, A. E., III. (2017). Caregiver Integration during discharge planning for older adults to reduce resource use: A meta-analysis. *Journal of the American Geriatric Society, 65*(8), 1748–1755. https://doi.org/10.1111/jgs.14873

Roter, D. L., Narayanan, S., Smith, K., Bullman, R., Rausch, P., Wolff, J. L., & Alexander, G. C. (2017). Family caregivers' facilitation of daily adult prescription medication use. *Patient and Education Counseling, 101*(5), 908–916. https://doi.org/10.1016/j.pec.2017.12.018

Sathitratanacheewin, S., Engelberg, R., Downey, L., Lee, R., Fausto, J., Starks, J., . . . Curtis, R. (2018). Temporal trends between 2010 and 2015 in intensity of care at end-of-lfie for patients with chronic illness: Influence of age under vs. over 65 years. *Journal of Pain and Symptom Management, 55*(1), 75–81. https://doi.org/10.1016/j.jpainsymman.2017.08.032

Schulz, R., Beach, S.R., Friedman, E., Martsolf, G., Rodakowski, J., & James, A. (2018). Changing structures and processes to support family caregivers of seriously ill patients. *Journal of Palliative Medicine, 21*(Suppl 2), S36–S42. https://doi.org/10.1093/geronb/gby021

Sharf, B., & Vanderford, M. L. (2003). Illness narratives and the social construction of health. In T. Thompson, A. Dorsey, K. Miller, & R. Parrot (Eds.), *Handbook of Health Communication* (pp. 9–34). Hillsdale, NJ: Lawrence Erlbaum.

Slater, S., Aoun, S., Hill, K., Walsh, D., Whitty, D., & Toye, C. (2019). Caregivers' experiences of a home support program after the hospital discharge of an older family member: A qualitative analysis. *BMC Health Services Research, 19,* 220. https://doi.org/10.1186/s12913-019-4042-0

Stall, N., Campbell, A., Reddy, M., & Rachon, P. (2019). Words matter: The language of family caregiving. *Journal of the American Geriatrics Society, 67,* 2008–2010. https://doi.org/10.1111/jgs.15988

Sterling, M. (2014). What family caregivers need from health IT and the healthcare system to be effective health managers. *Connected Health Resources*. Retrieved from www.connectedhealthresources.com

Stone, A. M., Mikucki-Enyart, S., Middleton, A., Caughlin, J. P., & Brown, L. E. (2012). Caring for a parent with lung cancer: Caregivers' perspectives on the role of communication. *Qualitative Health Research, 22*(7), 957–970. https://doi.org/10.1177/1049732312443428

Suitor, J. J., Gilligan, M., Johnson, K., & Pillemer, K. (2014). Caregiving perceptions of material favoritism, and tension among siblings. *Gerontologist, 54*(4), 580–588.

Sullivan, B.-J., Marcuccilli, L., Sloan, R., Gradus-Pizo, I., Bakas, T., Jung, M., & Pressler, S. (2016). Competence, compassion, and care of the self: Family caregiving needs and concerns in heart failure. *Journal of Cardiovascular Nursing, 31*(3), 209–214. https://doi.org/10.1097/JCN0000000000000241

Svendsboe, E., Terum, T., Testad, I., Aarsland, D., Ulstein, I., Corbett, A., & Rongve, A. (2016). Caregiver burden in family carers of people with dementia with Lewy bodies and Alzheimer's disease. *International Journal of Geriatric Psychiatry, 31*(9), 1075–1083.

Tao, H., McRoy, S., & Wang, L. (2017). Would mobile health be a solution to rehospitalization? *Nursing Health Science, 19*(2), 188–190. https://doi.org/10.1111/nhs.12330

Taylor, B. J., Irish, L. A., Martire, L. M., Siegle, G. J., Krafty, R. T., Schulz, R., & Hall, M. H. (2015). Avoidant coping and poor sleep efficiency in dementia caregivers. *Psychosomatic Medicine, 77*(9), 1050–1057.

Temel, J. S., Greer, J. A., Muzikansky, A., Gallagher, E. R., Admane, S., Jackson, V. A., . . . Lynch, T. J. (2010). Early palliative care for patients with metastatic non-small-cell lung cancer. *New England Journal of Medicine, 363*(8), 733–742. https://doi.org/10.1056/NEJMoa1000678

Thompson, C. M., Frisbie, A., Hudak, N., Okamoto, K. E., & Bell, S. (2017). "Understanding" as support for emerging adults whose parents have chronic health conditions: A life-span communication perspective. *Journal of Family Communication, 17*(4), 301–318.

Torres, H., Poorman, E., Tadepalli, U., Schoettler, C., Fung, C. H., Mushero, N., . . . McCormick, D. (2017). Coverage and access for Americans with chronic disease under the affordable care act: A quasi-experimental study. *Annals of Internal Medicine, 166*(7), 472–479. https://doi.org/10.7326/M16-1256

United Nations. (2019). *World population prospects 2019.* Retrieved from https://population.un.org/wpp/

US Department of Health and Human Services. (2018). *Quick guide to health literacy: Health literacy and health outcomes.* Retrieved from https://health.gov/communication/literacy/quickguide/factsliteracy.htm

Wakefield, B., & Vaughan-Sarrazin, M. (2018). Strain and satisfaction in caregivers of veterans with Type 2 Diabetes. *The Diabetes Educator, 44*(5), 435–443. https://doi.org/10.1177/0145721718790940

Wang, T., Molassiotis, A., Chung, B. P. M., & Tan, J. Y. (2018). Unmet care needs of advanced cancer patients and their informal caregivers: A systematic review. *BMC Palliative Care, 17*(1), 96. https://doi.org/10.1186/s12904-018-0346-9

Whitehead, L., Jacob, E., Towell, A., Abu-qamar, M., & Cole-Heath, A. (2017). The role of the family supporting the self-management of chronic conditions: A qualitative systematic review. *Journal of Clinical Nursing, 27*, 22–30. https://doi.org/10.1111/jocn.13775

Willes, K., Jagiello, K., Allen, M., & Motel, L. (2019). No matter what: A qualitative analysis of how LGBTQ families and allies define family through an interactive art project. *Journal of Family Communication, 19*(3), 277–289. https://doi.org/10.1080.15267431.2019.1632865

Wingham, J., Frost, J., Britten, N., Jolly, K., Greaves, C., Abraham, C., & Dalal, H. (2015). Needs of caregivers in heart failure management: A qualitative study. *Chronic Illness, 11*, 4. https://doi.org/10.1177/1742395315574765

Wittenberg, E., Borneman, T., Koczywas, M., Del Ferraro, C., & Ferrell, B. (2017). Cancer communication and family caregiver quality of life. *Behavioral Sciences (Basel), 7*(1), E12. https://doi.org/10.3390/bs7010012

Wittenberg, E., Goldsmith, J., & Kerr, A. (2019). Variation in health literacy among family caregiver communication types. *Psycho-Oncology, 28*(11), 2181–2187.

Wittenberg-Lyles, E., Goldsmith, J., Oliver, D. P., Demiris, G., Kruse, R. L., & Van Stee, S. (2013). Exploring oral literacy in communication with hospice caregivers. *Journal of Pain & Symptom Management, 46*(5), 731–736 https://doi.org/10.1016/j.jpainsymman.2012.11.006

Wittenberg-Lyles, E., Goldsmith, J., & Ragan, S. (2011). The shift to early palliative care: A typology of illness journeys and the role of nursing. *Clinical Journal of Oncology Nursing, 15*(3), 304–310. https://doi.org/10.1188/11.CJON.304-310

Wttenberg-Lyles, E., Goldsmith, J., Parker-Oliver, D., Demiris, G., & Rankin, A. (2012). Targeting communication interventions to decrease caregiver burden. *Seminars in Oncology Nursing, 28*(4), 262–270. https://doi.org/10.1016/j.soncn.2012.09.009

WHO CVD Risk Chart Working Group. (2019). World Health Organization cardiovascular disease risk charts: Revised models to estimate risk in 21 global regions. *The Lancet Global Health, 7*(10), E1332–E1345. https://doi.org/10.1016/S2214-109X(19)30318-3

Wu, J. R., Moser, D. K., DeWalt, D. A., Rayens, M. K., & Dracup, K. (2016). Health literacy mediates the relationship between age and health outcomes in patients with heart failure. *Circulation: Heart Failure, 9*(1), e002250. https://doi.org/10.1161/CIRCHEARTFAILURE.115.002250

Yuen, E., Knight, T., Ricciardelli, L. A., & Burney, S. (2018). Health literacy of caregivers of adult care recipients: A systematic scoping review. *Health & Social Care in the Community, 26*(2), e191–e206. https://doi.org/10.1111/hsc.12368

Zarit, S. H., Todd, P., & Zarit, J. M. (1986). Subjective burden of husbands and wives as caregivers: A longitudinal study. *Gerontologist, 26*(3), 260–266.

2

Health Literacy

The thing they never really did was interpret, sit and talk to us. We did get something written that says, shows abnormal increase in multiple areas, including the right scapula, multiple posterior and anterior ribs, multiple levels in the lumbar spine, the right wing and the left iliac. And we're talking to the new urologist and he's someone we've known for years, went to our church with us, and so Sam can talk to him. Get some questions kind of answered. We went and got another bone scan and are hoping we find someone who will talk to us about the scan. So, no one, so far, has interpreted the bone scans we got.

—Vera, wife of cancer patient Sam

Education level, socioeconomic status, occupation, race, literacy level. These are typical variables of concern and also of assumption when considering health literacy. Whatever the variables, *every* caregiver faces health literacy barriers. We believe that any caregiver navigating any chronic illness experiences caregiver communication burden related to these barriers. For Vera, she is missing an interpretation of results. Holding two master's degrees (one in public health) makes no difference to improving her health literacy—because she needs others to join with her to fill in the gaps. The missing pieces fall outside her ability to understand the status of her spouse's prostate cancer. Vera knows the medical names identifying her loved one's lytic bone tumors and readily uses that language at an 18th-grade level. But conceptual understanding is missing as no one has interpreted the scans; the communication burden of learning about and understanding these results is now heavily predicated on Vera's ability to communicate about caregiving.

Family caregiving requires a cache of complex communication and health literacy skills to navigate communication challenges. Essential to overcoming communication and health literacy barriers is understanding the family system in which communication patterns are produced. These patterns establish the ways in which family caregivers engage in communication about illness and are influenced by cultural and social contexts. This chapter describes how social determinants of health upon caregiving, the influence of culturally and linguistically appropriate language, and preferred language and language assistance availability influence health literacy needs. A palliative care approach addresses social conditions and cultural beliefs about illness and offers a better way to understand the role of the system, the provider, the family, and the community in shaping health literacy barriers and pathways for the caregiver. If caregivers are able to get what they need to support patient care, then patient care is likely to be improved and caregiver burden reduced.

HEALTH LITERACY IS CENTRAL TO FAMILY CAREGIVING

Yolanda: I had to be the one to change all the draining tube(s). And I wasn't for sure if I was doing it right, because I never went to a class. I was just thrown into this. It was like I never knew anything about cancer. I would go on the internet and just make sure I was doing the draining tubes right. I looked for what type of food that would help her. What to give her to help her iron, because she had iron deficiency. And she had to have blood transfusions twice under my care. If she had problems with anything, I would go to the Internet and look to see, should I call the doctor now? Should I take her to the hospital now?

In its origins and still today, health literacy has been viewed as the ability or inability of an *individual* to apply basic reading and numeracy skills to promote health or apply these skills in a healthcare situation (Ratzan & Parker, 2000; U.S. Department of Health and Human Services [USDHHS], Office of Disease Prevention and Health Promotion, 2010). Research and study of health literacy have produced additional definitions further broadening the idea to specifically include *communicate* as part of the concept. More recent definitions include "the degree to which an individual has the capacity to obtain, *communicate*, process, and understand health information and services in order to make appropriate health decisions" (Patient Protection and Affordable Care Act, 2010, p. 473) and "allows the public and personnel working in all health-related contexts to find, understand, evaluate, *communicate*, and use information" (Coleman et al., 2009, p. 1). The continuing evolution of the health literacy field has brought about new approaches with several viewing health literacy as a collaborative, dynamic, multidimensional, context-related proficiency that also conceptualizes the essential role of the healthcare provider and complex system demands that are placed upon patients and caregivers (Berkman et al., 2010; Parnell et al., 2019; Pleasant et al., 2016; Wittenberg et al., 2020).

As the demographic transformation occurs and the population continues to age, more and more adults will be relying upon caregivers for extended periods of time. Family caregivers will continue to serve as the foundation of the U.S. healthcare system and are necessary to support the increasing number of fragile elders and adults with disabilities (Family Caregiver Alliance, 2009). Caregivers require health literacy skills to adequately use health information when advocating for, understanding, communicating, and supporting chronically ill patients. Cancer caregivers, in particular, are charged with engaging in many conversations with multiple interdisciplinary healthcare providers regarding complex decisions over several stages of disease (Wittenberg et al., 2019). And although two thirds of chronic disease caregivers expressed that healthcare providers addressed their questions, less than half felt involved in conversations about health decisions, and a third shared that providers were not willing to discuss information with them (Michigan Medicine, University of Michigan, 2018). Provider resistance falls outside the skill set of the caregiver as an individual, underscoring the importance of including factors beyond the individual in understanding and improving health literacy.

Caregiver health literacy has been defined as the "personal characteristics and social resources needed for caregivers to access, understand, appraise, and use information and services to participate in decisions relating to the health and care of the recipient" (Yuen et al., 2014, p. 1471). Adequate health literacy skills are necessary for caregivers to participate in care and be a partner in decision-making (Rawlings & Tieman, 2015). A significant demand placed on caregivers of the acutely and chronically ill is the labor of communicating with members of the healthcare team and advocating for their care recipient.

Caregivers are often responsible for gathering and disseminating health information (Koehly et al., 2009) and accompanying patients to clinical visits (Wiles et al., 2018). Patients feel a sense of power when family members are involved in clinical visits (Arestedt et al., 2018), as family caregivers play a role in establishing mutual understanding between patient and healthcare provider (Arestedt et al., 2018). During clinical visits, caregivers work to improve the physician's understanding of the patient by introducing medical topics and clarifying or expanding medical information and history (Wolff et al., 2017). Caregivers are also tasked with sharing news of the diagnosis with others, another complex role that involves deciding what information should or can be shared, when to share it, whether they or the patient should give the news, and how news should be shared (Ewing et al., 2016). Health care providers report that caregivers listen, take notes, ask questions, and simplify information for the care recipient as well as supply providers with important patient medical information (Laidsaar-Powell et al., 2016).

In addition, the complex caregiver role includes assisting with and facilitating many medical activities, tasks, and treatments. While at first glance an activity may simply seem just that, we should be cognizant of the many different tasks involved in completing one activity. Rima Rudd, a senior lecturer on society and health literacy from Harvard School of Public Health, often speaks of "deconstructing" a health-related task and shared an example in an interview related to chronic disease management (Health Literacy Out Loud Podcast, 2009). She shared the activity example of giving a medication to a care recipient and how many components it takes to successfully complete this one activity. For example, the caregiver would have to obtain the prescription; go to the pharmacy or drug store; get the prescription filled; bring the medicine home; read, understand, and interpret the directions for taking the medicine; synthesize and differentiate this one medicine with all other medicines being taken; schedule the medicine by looking at times and days of week that the medicine is prescribed; track and monitor medicine schedules and side effects; keep track so the patient doesn't run out of the medicine; know how to request a refill if needed; and so on. You can get the gist of the number of varied tasks that are required just to take one medication. Caregivers need the skills and tools to accomplish each of the identified tasks in this one deconstructed example. Here two caregivers describe the activity of taking a medication but include unexpected complications that fall outside the bounds of this list of tasks that Rudd articulates.

> TONITA: Like yesterday, my mom, she took her pills regular that she take every day. But when she took her pain pills, which she take all the time, something happened. She was going into like—a zone out. And I was looking like, "Come on, let's go to the emergency room." I'm like, this is a normal, this normal. This what you take all the time. And all of a sudden I was like, you catching some kind of reaction. But I told her that probably she had been up trying to straighten up a little bit, and she sat straight down. I checked her blood pressure. It wasn't high. So I was like, I really don't know what else it could be. So it was confusing. Some of these medicines are so expensive. If she is taking a brand medicine, I guess I could check with the medicine manufacturers for additional help.
>
> TYRONE: Dad had this slight nausea. And the medication for nausea had such a big side effect. I had to make a decision, is relieving the nausea better than the side effects? And those decisions for a caregiver—am I equipped to be a caregiver?

In these caregiver reflections, vital caregiver skills and tools include the ability to read the prescription label, have access to transportation, feel empowered to ask healthcare providers or pharmacists for clarification, perform additional research, express needs and concerns, provide feedback, use a clock and calendar, develop reminder cues, measure, record or make a chart, and, the most significant skill—act in a crisis. All of these abilities are required for taking one medication! Multiply this for each medication a chronic illness patient may be taking, and then add all of the other caregiver responsibilities—it's no wonder that caregivers often feel burdened.

HEALTH LITERACY TAPESTRY AND NATIONAL ACTION PLAN TO SUPPORT CAREGIVERS

Health literacy related burden can be lessened if we are all part of the solution to foster systemwide efforts that seamlessly embed health literacy into all organizational missions, strategic plans, policies, and research and then assign accountability for all health literacy related activities. The National Action Plan to Improve Health Literacy (2010), a multisector effort, is based on the overarching principles that (a) everyone has the right to health information that helps them come to an informed decision and (b) all health services should be easy to understand for everyone and improve health and quality of life (USDHHS, Office of Disease Prevention and Health Promotion, 2010). The action plan suggests strategies for supporting patients and their caregivers based on seven goals listed in Box 2.1.

The Action Plan framework can be used to identify and address health literacy related barriers that can have a negative impact upon patient care (Baur, 2011) and the ability of caregivers to support care recipients. Viewing health literacy as a dynamic, multidimensional tapestry of diverse threads that embody an individual's life experiences and behaviors can also assist with reducing caregiver health literacy burdens and enhance communication, engagement, and activation (Parnell, 2015). The Health Literacy Tapestry (Figure 2.1) identifies three health literacy domains that represent how much a person understands what was said (oral communication), what was written (written communication), and what care and services are available and how to access them (environmental communication), (Parnell, 2015).

Box 2.1

NATIONAL ACTION PLAN TO IMPROVE HEALTH LITERACY

National Action Plan to Improve Health Literacy Goals

Goal 1   Develop and share accurate, accessible, actionable health and safety
         information
Goal 2   Promote health system changes to improve health information,
         communication, informed decision making and access
Goal 3   Incorporate accurate, standards-based, and developmentally
         appropriate health and science information and curricula in child care and
         education
Goal 4   Support and expand adult education, English language instruction, and
         culturally and linguistically appropriate health information
Goal 5   Build partnerships, develop guidance, and change policies
Goal 6   Increase research and development, implementation, and evaluation of
         practices and interventions to improve health literacy
Goal 7   Increase the dissemination and use of evidence-based health literacy
         practices and interventions

Source: U.S. Department of Health and Human Services, Office of Disease Prevention and Health Promotion. (2010). *National action plan to improve health literacy.* Washington, DC: Author, .

https://health.gov/our-work/health-literacy/national-action-plan-improve-health-literacy

---

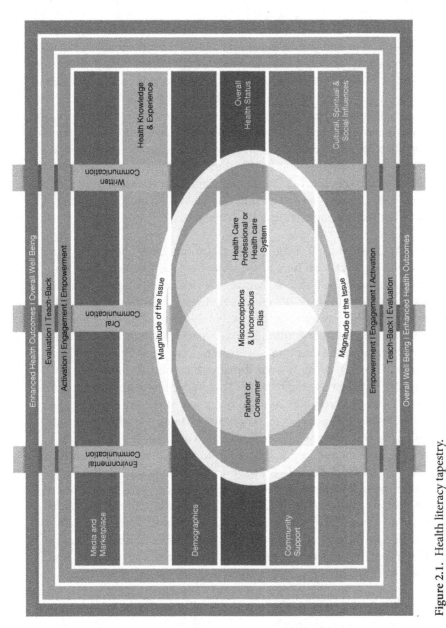

Figure 2.1. Health literacy tapestry.
SOURCE: Health Literacy in Nursing: Providing Person-Centered Care. Reprinted from T. A. Parnell, *Health literacy in nursing: Providing person-centered care*. New York: Springer, 2015. Reproduced with the permission of Springer Publishing Company, LLC.

Central to the Tapestry are the overlapping relationships between the patient/caregiver and the healthcare provider/system.

Together, the National Action Plan and the Health Literacy Tapestry offer several strategic suggestions to reduce health literacy barriers and support communication and caregivers. Goals 1, 2, and 7 of the Action Plan focus on promoting accurate, accessible, actionable health and safety information that improve access, communication and decision-making, and implementation of evidence-based health literacy practices and interventions (USDHHS, Office of Disease Prevention and Health Promotion, 2010). The Health Literacy Tapestry aligns with these goals by recognizing and honoring that each caregiver's demographics; health status and knowledge; exposure to health information through the media; prior health experience; and cultural, spiritual, and social influences present unique opportunities for providers to help reduce barriers to health literacy. In the following text, a caregiver describes the expertise required of her care for her spouse but also the emotional demands that complicate the tasks in her midst, further enforcing the idea that caregiver health literacy is a multidimensional accomplishment involving more than just the caregiver.

> Carolyn: You're scared you're going to do the wrong thing. I have to say, my husband, I have to stay on him all the time. Because if he gets more than a teaspoon of water, he'll drown. Because this is the only way. He doesn't breathe through his nose or his mouth. He breathes through that hole in his neck. And if he gets water in there, he could die. And so sometimes he doesn't wear this little cover thing in the shower, you know. So I have to worry about him all the time. I mean, I have to worry about him and I have to tell him, "Do this. Go clean your throat out. Drink water after you eat." You know, things like this. And he thinks I'm just nagging at him all the time, you know. Then you feel guilty. You feel guilty, you know. My whole life has changed. I'm the kind of person that's very active, and being with my friends and going here and there, you know? Jim's had to quit his job, you know. And so now, it's just him and me. And because he wants me to go everywhere with him. . . . [pause] I don't always want to go with him. But until he has, if he gets that prosthesis, he can get stopped up and go down in the back of his throat. Who is going to know what to do? Because with the kind of cancer he has, a lot of people don't know about neck and throat cancer. And there's a little plug. You have to put it in and rock it all the way at the back so he can breathe. If you don't do that, he's dead. So constantly that's on my mind. And you don't want to talk to your family about it.

In the role of family caregiver, communication with family is a significant stress that contributes to caregiver burden (Wittenberg-Lyles et al., 2012). Health care information can vary along a chronic illness continuum of care in amount, timing, and style. Both care recipient and caregiver will be interacting with many different healthcare providers and settings. Caregivers might come across print health information or instructions, medication demands and contraindications, diagnosis or prognosis information, interpretation of vital signs, and even treatment choices. In each step along the way, the caregiver is put in a position of communicating with the healthcare providers and staff as well as with the care recipient, which presents challenging communicative relationships to monitor and manage. Health literacy related barriers can impact willingness to discuss or complete advance directives and has also been associated with poorer pain management, medication errors, and nonadherence to the treatment plan by the care recipient or their family caregiver (Wittenberg et al., 2015).

An additional component that is represented in the Health Literacy Tapestry model is the thread dedicated to community support. The focal point of Action Plan goals 3 and 4 is the *community*. The community setting is where many people learn how to access health information and services. This can include not only school, adult education, childcare, and library and literacy programs (Baur, 2011) but also extends to less formal community structures and identities such as church, neighborhood areas, common identifications (e.g., parents of those with cancer), and support groups. Trust about treatment decisions and health information can be highest between caregivers and community, as compared to caregivers and providers or caregivers and family (Terui et al., 2020).

Goal 5 includes building partnerships and also developing guidance and policy change (USDHHS, Office of Disease Prevention and Health Promotion, 2010). Healthcare providers can offer critical insight and experience to other providers in a collaborative fashion. The process, lessons learned, and outcomes of these partnerships can inform future projects with other providers, in other health systems, and with new provider-partners. Goal 6 is central to increasing health literacy research, implementation, and evaluation of practices and approaches to enhance health literacy (USDHHS, Office of Disease Prevention and Health Promotion, 2010).

SOCIAL DETERMINANTS AND HEALTH LITERACY

Health literacy is associated with social determinants of health and with health outcomes (Logan et al., 2015). The conditions in which people are born, grow, live, work, and play are collectively referred to as social determinants of health and include the structures that shape the conditions of daily life (Bennett et al., 2018; World Health Organization, 2019). More simply, social determinants of health are the shared nonmedical factors that can contribute to a person's general health, ability to function, and overall quality of life.

The six common social determinants of health domains are economic stability, physical environment and neighborhood, education, food, social and community support, and the healthcare system (Bennett et al., 2018). The influence of social determinants of health upon health outcomes such as poverty, living environment, educational level (Sorensen et al., 2012) and homelessness (Olshansky, 2017) has been widely reported. Although providers have historically focused on making a diagnosis and developing a treatment plan for a patient's clinical disease(s), they are beginning to take a more holistic, person-centered approach to patient care and treatment options that recognize the whole person experiencing the illness. Realizing social determinants of health is essential for improving health outcomes such as mortality, morbidity, life expectancy, health care status, and functional limitations (Healthy People 2020, 2019).

Individuals with more health literacy barriers experience more hospitalizations, greater use of emergency care, less adherence to treatment recommendations, worse health status, and higher mortality rates (Berkman et al., 2011). Akin to the social determinants of health, low health literacy skills also contribute to similar health inequities and poor health outcomes. Although every caregiver is likely to experience low health literacy at various times, low health literacy disproportionately impacts racial and ethnic minorities, persons with limited English proficiency (LEP), older adults, and those with less education and lower socioeconomic status (USDHHS, Office of Disease Prevention and Health Promotion, 2010). The expanding science tells us that caregivers with less engaged/available elements of providers, community, family, and health systems face bigger barriers. Caregivers who have fewer resources and points of access are in a position to rely predominantly on their individual skills without regularly supportive and involved relational efforts; this impacts a caregiver's ability to provide a strong health literacy network, which builds the architecture for quality patient care and outcomes.

Caregivers managing chronic illness for care recipients can face many health literacy–related burdens. Caregivers can serve as mediator and interpreter between the care recipient and the healthcare provider (Arestedt et al., 2018). For many, increased understanding comes from having key parties present in the clinical visit, as shared discussions among the patient, caregiver, and provider can make it easier to discuss illness, treatment, and self-care and can strengthen relationships. Caregivers who attend appointments with patients receive more time and attention from healthcare professionals. To help patients understand aspects of their care, caregivers often repeat explanations, reframe information in plain language form, and ask questions to resolve confusion and worry (Washington et al., 2019).

Culturally and Linguistically Appropriate Standards

All cultures have traditions and beliefs about illness and treatment that are generationally passed on; caregiving is a central aspect to relationships between loved ones and how family members perform and show that they belong to one another (Kleinman, 2012). Caregivers may experience incredible burden when caring for recipients with chronic or serious illness, and the challenges can become more colossal and overwhelming when there are cultural or linguistic disparities. An individual's culture is a reflection of group values, beliefs, and behaviors that are influenced by cultural and social contexts.

Cultural factors influence family involvement (Laidsaar-Powell et al., 2016) and may result in a limited desire or ability to participate in treatment decision-making, misunderstanding of disease, less desire/need for information, inaccurate assessment of risk, and fewer questions asked of healthcare providers (Campesino et al., 2012; Costas-Muniz et al., 2013; Mead et al., 2013). These factors include level of acculturation and language (Mead et al., 2013), LEP (Campesino et al., 2012; Costas-Muniz et al., 2013), use of translators (Costas-Muniz et al., 2013), lack of available educational materials in languages other than monolingual English or bilingual English/Spanish (Costas-Muniz et al., 2013), and health beliefs. When family members don't possess a shared understanding of the illness, they tend to avoid the healthcare system and the person with the illness (Arestedt et al., 2018).

The Enhanced National Standards for Culturally and Linguistically Appropriate Services (CLAS) in Health and Health Care (the National CLAS Standards) is a framework that outlines standards for caring for the nation's increasingly diverse communities. The overarching standard is to "provide effective, equitable, under-standable and respectful quality care and services that are responsive to diverse cultural health beliefs and practices, preferred languages, health literacy and other communication needs" (USDHHS, Office of Minority Health, 2016). As seen in Box 2.2, the three main themes of the CLAS standards are governance, leadership and workforce; communication and language assistance; and engagement, con-tinuous improvement, and accountability.

Preferred Language and Language Assistance Services

Stress and difficulty contribute to caregiver communication burden when English is not the caregiver/patient's preferred language. As per the U.S. Census Bureau, the term limited English proficiency (LEP) refers to any person over the age of 5 years who has a limited ability to read, speak, write, or understand the English language (Zong & Batalova, 2015). The LEP population has grown 80% between 1990 and 2013, from 14 million to 25 million; has completed less ed-ucation; and is more likely to have lower socioeconomic status when compared to English-proficient populations (Zong & Batalova, 2015). For LEP caregivers, communicating clearly with healthcare providers in their preferred language is necessary for them to fully participate and advocate for safe, meaningful access to quality health information and services.

A language difference should not be the factor that keeps a patient/care-giver from health information. Health literacy is not limited to reading alone, but also includes writing, listening, speaking, numeracy skills, critical thinking, decision-making, and cultural sensitivity abilities—not just for the patient, but also for the family caregiver, providers, and healthcare systems (Goldsmith & Terui, 2018). The connection between literacy and culture is inextricable. What patients/families face in healthcare settings explains a great deal of the health lit-eracy load, in addition to cultural barriers that can reduce success in care. Many times there is a simple overestimation of patient/family ability to absorb termi-nology (i.e., aural literacy demand), make sense of rare words, or stay focused in the midst of words and ideas that invite communication burden (Koch-Weser et al., 2010).

Box 2.2

The Enhanced National Standards for Culturally and Linguistically Appropriate Services in Health and Health Care (National CLAS Standards)

Principal Standard

1. Provide effective, equitable, understandable, and respectful quality care and services that are responsive to diverse cultural health beliefs and practices, preferred languages, health literacy, and other communication needs.

Governance, Leadership, and Workforce

2. Advance and sustain organizational governance and leadership that promotes CLAS and health equity through policy, practices, and allocated resources.
3. Recruit, promote, and support a culturally and linguistically diverse governance, leadership, and workforce that are responsive to the population in the service area.
4. Educate and train governance, leadership, and workforce in culturally and linguistically appropriate policies and practices on an ongoing basis.

Communication and Language Assistance

5. Offer language assistance to individuals who have limited English proficiency and/ or other communication needs, at no cost to them, to facilitate timely access to all healthcare and services.
6. Inform all individuals of the availability of language assistance services clearly and in their preferred language, verbally and in writing.
7. Ensure the competence of individuals providing language assistance, recognizing that the use of untrained individuals and/or minors as interpreters should be avoided.
8. Provide easy-to-understand print and multimedia materials and signage in the languages commonly used by the populations in the service area.

Engagement, Continuous Improvement, and Accountability

9. Establish culturally and linguistically appropriate goals, policies, and management accountability, and infuse them throughout the organization's planning and operations.
10. Conduct ongoing assessments of the organization's CLAS-related activities and integrate CLAS-related measures into measurement and continuous quality improvement activities.
11. Collect and maintain accurate and reliable demographic data to monitor and evaluate the impact of CLAS on health equity and outcomes and to inform service delivery.
12. Conduct regular assessments of community health assets and needs and use the results to plan and implement services that respond to the cultural and linguistic diversity of populations in the service area.

13. Partner with the community to design, implement, and evaluate policies, practices, and services to ensure cultural and linguistic appropriateness.
14. Create conflict and grievance resolution processes that are culturally and linguistically appropriate to identify, prevent, and resolve conflicts or complaints.
15. Communicate the organization's progress in implementing and sustaining CLAS to all stakeholders, constituents, and the general public.

Source: U.S. Department of Health and Human Services, Office of Minority Health. (2016). *National standards for culturally and linguistically appropriate services in health and health care: Compendium of state-sponsored national CLAS standards implementation activities.* Washington, DC: Author.

PALLIATIVE CARE AND HEALTH LITERACY

A palliative care approach offers a better way to understand health literacy barriers by addressing the ways that an individual's cultural and linguistic preferences influence decisions regarding chronic disease management. Palliative care is a form of medicine that is offered simultaneously with all other appropriate (curative or noncurative) medical treatments and thus is for all patients of any age suffering from stressful, painful, or debilitating symptoms (see Chapter 3 of this volume). In palliative care, the patient and family are seen as one, and the physical, psychological, social, and spiritual suffering that accompanies disease is addressed by valuing communication critical to these topics. Palliative care acknowledges the unique role of family caregivers and emphasizes a triadic communication process in illness that involves the patient, family caregiver, and healthcare team. In fact, communication is considered a significant modality of clinical work in palliative care—making it the only area of medical care that prioritizes communication so substantially.

A palliative care approach to chronic illness involves communication aimed at helping the patient and family understand the disease and disease trajectory, including end-of-life care. Differences in beliefs about treatment and issues related to dying or end of life can be especially complex for culturally and linguistically diverse patients and caregivers and their providers (Kirby et al., 2018). Communication about treatment plans, medication management, shared decision-making, and end-of-life issues are more challenging across language barriers. Language barriers can influence symptom assessment, use of hospice services, health quality, and outcomes of LEP individuals at end of life (Silva et al., 2016).

Complex, accurate, and highly sensitive conversations about palliative care and end of life cannot occur without supportive language services (Schenker et al., 2012). When there is a difference in the preferred language of a caregiver or care recipient and the healthcare provider, it is essential that a professional medical interpreter be used to communicate linguistically and culturally accurate information (National Consensus Project for Quality Palliative Care, 2018). Use of a professional medical interpreter meets the legal requirements of Title VI of the Civil Rights Act and should be offered to all patients and caregivers with LEP (Juckett & Unger, 2014).

> Kanda, a 30-year-old woman who had just come to the United States from Bangkok, and her husband Dusit, 40 years old, had been living in the United States for eight years and were expecting their first child. Doctors and nurses told them their baby's brain was very irregular in its appearance. Kanda went into early labor and delivered at 26 weeks. Their daughter had a microcephalic brain.
>
> Kanda and Dusit's baby was placed in the neonatal intensive care unit, and they were told that their baby girl would need a lot of care and intervention, and her life expectancy was unknown. Providers told the parents that their baby would be made comfortable, but there was little else that medicine could offer. A neonatal intensive care unit nurse drew a picture of the brain with its areas to show the couple how their daughter's was incomplete. Dusit was shocked, stating that he could not believe his baby was so unwell.
>
> The two stunned parents did not know that they had the right to an interpreter and the responsibility to ask questions of their care providers. The two of them were very limited in their English proficiency and had been raised in a collectivistic culture. They struggled to understand their child's prognosis and early arrival. Their exposure to physicians and nurses in Bangkok had been limited. They felt truly lost without their family around to help them understand and face the hours and days ahead.

Do these parents really understand what is happening to their child? What kinds of planning and intervention might have been effective with this family to help increase their health literacy? Caregivers commonly assume the role of interpreter in medical situations (Gray et al., 2011); however, this can bring additional communication challenges. Errors in medical interpretation are common, especially with the use of an ad hoc interpreter such as a family member or caregiver interpreter (Wolters Kluwer Health: Lippincott Williams and Wilkins, 2015).

Information conveyed by the interpreting caregiver can be mediated and culturally variable. Certain words such as *survival, comfortable,* or *hospice* will have different meanings or associations across varying cultural contexts. Interpreting caregivers may also be unwilling to speak about dying or end of life as it may not be part of their cultural beliefs or may be viewed as a weakness (Kirby et al., 2018). This may result in misinformation, confusion, frustration, and errors during the interpretation process for the clinician, patient and caregiver. A dramatic account of the need for "cultural brokers"—those people who can translate both linguistic and cultural differences—was journalist Anne Fadiman's book *The Spirit Catches You and You Fall Down* (Fadiman, 1997), which relates the story of a Hmong child in California. Medical anthropologist Arthur Kleinman also speaks of this need in several of his works (Kleinman, 1988, 2012).

There are differences for racial and ethnic populations involving palliative care, commonly associated with end-of-life care. Underuse of palliative care services is due to mistrust of the American health system, differences in perception, lack of knowledge about disease trajectory, preference for life-prolonging treatment regardless of a poor outcome, and religious beliefs (Cain et al., 2018). When in the midst of care that offers palliative services, chronically ill racial/ethnic minorities are less engaged with these services (Cunningham et al., 2017). When professional interpreters are not used to assist with the introduction of palliative care services, LEP patients experience worse quality of end-of-life care (Silva et al., 2016). When there are language barriers among care recipients, caregivers, and healthcare providers, accurate discussions about pain, chronic illness, symptoms, or end of life become less productive (Roat, 2012). Greater attention is needed to acknowledge each person's diversity, especially in regard to cultural, linguistic, and spiritual values and beliefs and to appreciate the unique nature of each patient–caregiver–provider partnership.

CAREGIVER COMMUNICATION PATTERNS AND CAREGIVER HEALTH LITERACY SKILLS

A caregiver's background, education, economic stability, physical environment, family, community, and healthcare system access give rise to health literacy barriers and pathways. These social and cultural factors also influence communication patterns for family caregivers that contribute to the ways in which they communicate about chronic illness. When communication about illness within the family is difficult for the caregiver, communication with healthcare providers and staff may also be difficult. Decisions about treatment, goals of care, and end-of-life care are not only dependent upon the caregiver's health literacy skills, but these decisions are also predicated upon the caregiver's ability to communicate with the patient, family, and healthcare providers and can contribute to communication burden.

Variance in social and cultural factors produce a wide range of communication abilities and health literacy barriers for caregivers. If the caregiver is adept at organizing and very task oriented, perhaps a strength would be that she is able to plan for and schedule upcoming appointments, food delivery, or medication refills. On the other hand, if she lives in an urban community and does not have a car or driver's license, an area of need will be transportation to and from appointments, tests, and procedures. Or, if caregivers find it tough to advocate, speak up, and communicate, perhaps they can enlist the help of another family member or friend who finds this easier when attending appointments or hospital visits. The overlapping relationship between patient/caregiver and the healthcare provider/ system create health literacy challenges that result in more communication difficulty with providers and increased communication burden (Fields et al., 2018).

Health literacy has historically been focused on an individual's skills, or lack thereof, to obtain, process, and understand basic health information and services

(Berkman et al., 2010). But health literacy has evolved to more accurately represent the complex and multidimensional aspect of healthcare and more recently has been defined as a

> dynamic, collaborative and mutually beneficial proficiency incorporating prior health knowledge and experience, individual characteristics, health status, cultural and linguistic preferences, and cognitive abilities influencing the ability of organizations, *caregivers*, and healthcare recipients to access, understand, and use health information and services to make informed actionable decisions and enhance health outcomes. (Parnell et al., 2019, p. 8)

This updated definition heightened attention to the essential and expanding role of the caregiver. We know now that the labors of achieving health literacy become even greater a burden for individuals with low socioeconomic status and low educational achievements (Denning & DiNenno, 2017). However, we believe that interactions are *co-constructed* by those engaged in the interaction, and thus health literacy is a multidimensional, group effort.

Health literacy involves not only caregivers' and patients' cognitive and functional skills, but also the collaborative efforts between patients, caregivers, healthcare organizations, healthcare providers, and communities (Batterham et al., 2016; Chou et al., 2015). This collaborative view of health literacy underscores the synergy between healthcare recipients, formal and informal healthcare providers, and resources from healthcare systems to reduce health literacy barriers, ease communication burden, and lessen inequities in health.

OUR CAREGIVERS AND HEALTH LITERACY

We want to return to our four family caregivers from Chapter 1. These narratives illustrate further dimensions of these caregivers to reveal caregiving communication challenges related to health literacy barriers.

Maggie Burkhart

As a very little girl she knew that her parents drank a lot. Alcohol was heavily in her midst for half of the day, every day. Her dad was the heavier drinker though, even behaving explosively in the late evenings after the rest of the house had quieted. The louder, more raucous nights were predictable by Maggie and her siblings based on whether her Dad would eat dinner or not. The less he ate for dinner, the more drunk he became. Their mom was not able to stifle his habits and often joined him in a less extreme version of overconsumption. For Maggie, she learned early how to avoid the easy pitfalls in communicating with heavily inebriated adults—be quiet, organized, as far away as possible, agreeable, and, most of all, help with things like dishes, laundry, and cleaning. But do it as quietly as possible.

Her oldest brother, Billy, was a decade her senior. He was often gone and not a regular presence in the household. In his mid-teens, he became a member of a very successful band that would find and still enjoys an international audience, awards, and fame. Billy mirrored his Dad's coping behavior with alcohol. But his lifestyle did not require him to get up and work each day, provide for children, and appear to be a high-functioning citizen of his local community. And so he drank heavily. And Maggie, the youngest, knew the mantra of "We need to protect Billy" well, and like her other family members, Maggie held fast to that notion throughout life.

In their early 50s, with the children grown and gone, Maggie's parents stopped drinking. Her mom declared no more alcohol in the home and demanded Maggie's dad leave if he didn't stop drinking. And so they both stopped and tell the story as though it happened in one moment and neither looked back or experienced temptation into their addictions after this. That's how the story goes.

Sharon Jenks

The first 30 years of her life were lived in poverty. She grew up with her granny as her primary caretaker. Along with two sisters, they lived in a two-bedroom apartment near the city center. Each girl shared the same mom but different dads. Their mom was intermittently present, even living with them on and off. But Granny was their stability. She herself worked at a nearby grocery market, a job she had held for as long as Sharon could remember. The girls took the city bus to school. Only Sharon graduated from high school.

She moved out upon graduation and immediately married. She never returned to school. Her three boys came in rapid succession. She cared for them as she had not been cared for, and once they were school-aged she sought employment. Not having further education beyond high school never deterred her efforts. Her interpersonal skills and will to achieve impressed a legal office. She began work as a receptionist.

Through her life, she had been surrounded by pretty healthy people. Also, she had never had health care or access to a health system. During her childhood, she had no memory of seeing a healthcare provider or of her granny seeing a provider. Care for her own children was limited to required shots for school. She had survived an incredibly economically depressed childhood with little adult support, and now in adulthood and with her children healthy and nearly grown, she was moving into a more powerful position at the legal office and also embracing the reality that she loved her husband but in her deepest self knew that she was a lesbian.

Estella Rodriguez

Her first recollection of translating for her parents in a doctor's office was before her brother Melvin was born. Her mom went to the doctor one time before he arrived, and she was *very* pregnant, as Estella recalled. It was just Estella and her mom. At the tender age of six, Estella was the family spokesperson when it came to English. Born of Spanish-speaking parents, Estella was exposed to English in school. Her parents had been in Texas for almost 10 years but were not and never would be comfortable speaking English. Estella, the eldest child, would eventually have a total of three younger siblings. The same family practitioner's office would be a fixture in their lives until her parents retired and moved to a different community. Estella became familiar with the two physicians running the clinic, and over time they would not only expect to see her with her mom or dad and brothers and sister, but they would rely on and thank her for her bilingual abilities. Even after Estella was an adult with her own children, she would still attend her mom's appointments to serve as translator, as would her siblings if they were available. Never was a trained interpreter offered to the family.

When Estella was in seventh grade, she went with her mom to the doctor. Not until she was sitting in the office with the physician did Estella learn why they were there. Without expressing emotion, her Mom stoically described bleeding and cramping heavily; the then-12-year old Estella did her best to translate Spanish to English. Until this moment, Estella had not known that her mom was pregnant and may have lost the baby. The doctor administered a pregnancy test to check for viability. While they waited on their own in the office, her mom began to cry. Estella squeezed back one tear after the next, patting her mom's hand while they waited to hear the results.

Viv Gray

It was clear that she was a disappointment to her parents, for whatever reason. From the outside looking in, the disappointment she felt and experienced did not make much sense. Over time, she shared less and less about her hopes and plans and endeavors, simply to have less interaction with this pall of disappointment—not just from her parents but also her siblings. In many respects, Viv was an introvert and would solve problems and process difficulties on her own. The family was simply not a place to unpack difficulties and uncertainties.

Her most intimate connections were with friends, co-workers, and especially now with Jake. They were on their own as a couple. But they were a stalwart and deeply loving unit. They sort of grew up together, in the same town and school with many of the same friends. They shared a close admiration for one another. Jake was smart and nerdy and offered Viv an interesting perspective on life in her teens.

To her surprise, Jake committed to the military at the conclusion of high school as a way to pay for college, and she wouldn't see him for four years. They briefly connected in Viv's senior year of college, but it would be another two decades before they would fully commit to their friendship and care for each other. Viv knew that Jake was in Desert Storm. She heard stories from their mutual friends that he had suffered frost bite and lost toes and had great difficulties with posttraumatic stress disorder, but she had no real sense of the impact of his military duty on his health and how these issues would evolve.

Viv was smart, creative and intuitive and able to navigate just about any jam. Her travels and turns in life sealed these abilities. She had an orientation to health-care mostly through her own work in a veterinary clinic. But she had never had to care for a person or a family member. This was about to change.

REFERENCES

Arestedt, L., Persson, C., Ramgard, M., & Benzein, E. (2018). Experiences of encounters with healthcare professionals through the lenses of families living with chronic illness. *Journal of Clinical Nursing, 27*(3–4), 836–847. https://doi.org/10.1111/jocn.14126

Batterham, R. W., Hawkins, M., Collins, P. A., Buchbinder, R., & Osborne, R. H. (2016). Health literacy: Applying current concepts to improve health services and reduce health inequalities. *Public Health, 132*, 3–12. https://doi.org/http://dx.doi.org/10.1016/j.puhe.2016.01.001

Baur, C. (2011). Calling the nation to act: Implementing the national action plan to improve health literacy. *Nursing Outlook, 59*(2), 63–69. https://doi.org/10.1016/j.outlook.2010.12.003

Bennett, N. M., Brown, M. T., Green, T., Hall, L. L., & Winkler, A. M. (2018, August 30). Addressing social determinants of health (SDOH): Beyond the clinic walls. *American Medical Association*. Retrieved from https://edhub.ama-assn.org/steps-forward/module/2702762

Berkman, N. D., Davis, T. C., & McCormack, L. (2010). Health literacy: What is it? *Journal of Health Communication, 15*(Suppl 2), 9–19. https://doi.org/10.1080/10810730.2010.499985

Berkman, N. D., Sheridan, S. L., Donahue, K. E., Halpern, D. J., & Crotty, K. (2011). Low health literacy and health outcomes: An updated systematic review. *Annals of Internal Medicine, 155*(2), 97–107. https://doi.org/10.7326/0003-4819-155-2-201107190-00005

Cain, C. L., Surbone, A., Elk, R., & Kagawa-Singer, M. (2018). Culture and palliative care: Preferences, communication, meaning, and mutual decision making. *Journal of Pain & Symptom Management, 55*(5), 1408–1419. https://doi.org/10.1016/j.jpainsymman.2018.01.007

Campesino, M., Saenz, D. S., Choi, M., & Krouse, R. S. (2012). Perceived discrimination and ethnic identity among breast cancer survivors. *Oncology Nursing Forum, 39*(2), E91–E100. https://doi.org/10.1188/12.ONF.E91-E100

Chou, W. S., Gaysynsky, A., & Persoskie, A. (2015). Health literacy and communication in palliative care. In E. Wittenberg, B. R. Ferrell, J. Goldsmith, T. Smith, S. L. Ragan, M. Glajchen, & G. Handzo (Eds.), *Textbook of palliative care communication* (pp. 90–101). New York, NY: Oxford University Press.

Coleman, C. S., Kurtz-Rossi, J., McKinney, A., Pleasant, I., Rootman, L., & Shohet, L. (2009). *The Calgary charter on health literacy*. Montreal, QB: Centre for Literacy.

Costas-Muniz, R., Sen, R., Leng, J., Aragones, A., Ramirez, J., & Gany, F. (2013). Cancer stage knowledge and desire for information: Mismatch in Latino cancer patients? *Journal of Cancer Education, 28*(3), 458–465. https://doi.org/10.1007/s13187-013-0487-8

Cunningham, T. J., Croft, J. B., Liu, Y., Lu, H., Eke, P. I., & Giles, W. H. (2017). Vital signs: Racial disparities in age-specific mortality among Blacks or African Americans—United States, 1999–2015. *MMWR, 66*(17), 444–456. https://doi.org/10.15585/mmwr.mm6617e1

Denning, P., & DiNenno, E. (2017). Communities in crisis: Is there a generalized HIV epidemic in impoverished urban areas of the United States? *Center for Disease Control and Prevention.* Retrieved from https://www.cdc.gov/hiv/group/poverty.html

Ewing, G., Ngwenya, N., Benson, J., Gilligan, D., Bailey, S., Seymour, J., & Farquhar, M. (2016). Sharing news of a lung cancer diagnosis with adult family members and friends: A qualitative study to inform a supportive intervention. *Patient Education & Counseling, 99*(3), 378–385. https://doi.org/10.1016/j.pec.2015.09.013

Fadiman, A. (1997). *The spirit catches you and you fall down.* New York, NY: MacMillan.

Family Caregiver Alliance. (2009). *Caregiving.* Retrieved from https://www.caregiver.org/caregiving

Fields, B., Rodakawski, J., Everette, J. A., & Beach, S. (2018). Caregiver health literacy predicting healthcare communication and system navigation difficulty. *American Psychological Association, 36*(4), 482–492. https://doi.org/10.1037/fsh0000368

Goldsmith, J., & Terui, S. (2018). Family oncology caregivers and relational health literacy. *Challenges, 9*(35), 1–10. https://doi.org/10.3390/challe9020035

Gray, B., Hilder, J., & Donaldson, H. (2011). Why do we not use trained interpreters for all patients with limited English proficiency? Is there a place for using family members? *Australian Journal of Primary Health, 17,* 240–249.

Health Literacy Out Loud Podcast. (2009). *Dr. Rima Rudd talks about the health literacy burden in healthcare (HLOL #15).* Retrieved from https://healthliteracy.com/2009/05/04/dr-rima-rudd-talks-about-the-health-literacy-burden-in-healthcare-hlol-15/

Healthy People 2020. (2019). *2020 topics and objectives: Social determinants of health.* Retrieved from https://www.healthypeople.gov/2020/topics-objectives/topic/social-determinants-of-health

Juckett, G., & Unger, K. (2014). Appropriate us of medical interpreters. *American Family Physician, 90*(7), 476–480.

Kirby, E., Lwin, Z., Kenny, K., Broom, A., Birman, H., & Good, P. (2018). "It doesn't exist . . .": Negotiating palliative care from a culturally and linguistically diverse patient and caregiver perspective. *BMC Palliative Care, 17*(1), 90. https://doi.org/10.1186/s12904-018-0343-z

Kleinman, A. (1988). *The illness narratives: Suffering, healing, and the human condition.* New York, NY: Basic Books.

Kleinman, A. (2012). Caregiving as moral experience. *The Lancet, 380*(9853), 1550–1551. https://doi.org/https://doi.org/10.1016/S0140-6736(12)61870-4

Koch-Weser, S., Rudd, R., & DeJong, W. (2010). Quantifying word use to study health literacy in doctor–patient communication. *Journal of Health Communication, 15,* 590–602. https://doi.org/10.1080/10810730.2010.499592

Koehly, L. M., Peters, J. A., Kenen, R., Hoskins, L. M., Ersig, A. L., Kuhn, N. R., . . . Greene, M. H. (2009). Characteristics of health information gatherers, disseminators, and blockers within families at risk of hereditary cancer: Implications for family health communication interventions. *American Journal of Public Health, 99*(12), 2203–2209. doi:10.2105/AJPH.2008.154096

Laidsaar-Powell, R., Butow, P., Bu, S., Charles, C., Gafni, A., . . . Juraskova, I. (2016). Family involvement in cancer treatment decision-making: A qualitative study of patient, family, and clinician attitudes and experiences. *Patient Education & Counseling, 99*(7), 1146–1155. https://doi.org/10.1016/j.pec.2016.01.014

Logan, R. A., Wong, W. F., Villaire, M., Daus, G., Parnell, T. A., Willis, E., & Paasche-Orlow, M. (2015). *Health literacy: A necessary element for achieving health equity (Discussion paper).* doi:10.31478/201507a

Mead, E. L., Doorenbos, A. Z., Javid, S. H., Haozous, E. A., Alvord, L. A., Flum, D. R., & Morris, A. M. (2013). Shared decision-making for cancer care among racial and ethnic minorities: A systematic review. *American Journal of Public Health, 103*(12), e15–e29. https://doi.org/10.2105/AJPH.2013.301631

Michigan Medicine, University of Michigan. (2018, January 16). In chronic disease care, family helpers are key, but feel left out. *Science Daily.* Retrieved from www.sciencedaily.com/releases/2018/01/180116123950.htm

National Consensus Project for Quality Palliative Care. (2018). *Clinical practice guidelines for quality palliative care.* https://www.nationalcoalitionhpc.org/ncp

Olshansky, E. F. (2017). Social determinants of health: The role of nursing. *American Journal of Nursing, 117*(12), 11. https://doi.org/10.1097/01.NAJ.0000527463.16094.39

Parnell, T. A. (2015). *Health literacy in nursing: Providing person-centered care.* New York, NY: Springer.

Parnell, T. A., Stichler, J. F., Barton, A. J., Loan, L. A., Boyle, D. K., & Allen, P. E. (2019). A concept analysis of health literacy. *Nursing Forum, 54*(3), 315–327. https://doi.org/10.1111/nuf.12331

Patient Protection and Affordable Care Act, 42 U.S.C. § 18001 (2010).

Pleasant, A., Rudd, R., O'Leary, C., Paasche-Orlow, M., Allen, M. P., Alvarado-Little, W., . . . Rosen, S. (2016, April 4). *Considerations for a new definition of health literacy (Discussion paper).* Retrieved from https://nam.edu/considerations-for-a-new-definition-of-health-literacy/

Ratzan, S., & Parker, R. M. (2000). Introduction. In C. Selden, M. Zorn, S. Ratzan, & R. M. Parker (Eds.), *National Library of Medicine current bibliographies in medicine* (Health Literacy NLM pub. no. CBM 2000-1). Washington, DC: National Institutes of Health, U.S. Department of Health and Human Services.

Rawlings, D., & Tieman, J. (2015). Patient and career information: Can they read and understand it? An example from palliative care. *Australian Nursing and Midwifery Journal, 23*(5), 26–29.

Roat, C. (2012). Language lessons: Palliative care training for interpreters (Issue brief). *California Healthcare Foundation.* Retrieved from https://www.chcf.org/wp-content/uploads/2017/12/PDF-LanguageLessonsPalliativeCareTrainingforInterpreters.pdf

Schenker, Y., Smith, A. K., Arnold, R. M., & Fernandez, A. (2012). "Her husband doesn't speak much English": Conducting a family meeting with an interpreter. *Journal of Palliative Medicine, 15*(4), 494–498. https://doi.org/10.1089/jpm.2011.0169

Silva, M. D., Genoff, M., Zaballa, A., Jewell, S., Stabler, S., Gany, F. M., & Diamond, L. C. (2016). Interpreting at the end of life: A systematic review of the impact of interpreters on the delivery of palliative care services to cancer patients with limited

English proficiency. *Journal of Pain & Symptom Management, 51*(3), 569–580. https://doi.org/10.1016/j.jpainsymman.2015.10.011

Sorensen, K., Van den Broucke, S., Fullam, J., Doyle, G., Pelikan, J., Slonska, Z., & Brand, H. (2012). Health literacy and public health: A systematic review and integration of definitions and models. *BMC Public Health, 12*, 80. https://doi.org/10.1186/1471-2458-12-80

Terui, S., Goldsmith, J., Huang, J., & Williams, J. (2020). Health literacy and health communication training for underserved patients and informal family caregivers. *Journal of Health Care for the Poor and Underserved,* 31, 635–645.

U.S. Department of Health and Human Services, Office of Disease Prevention and Health Promotion. (2010). *National action plan to improve health literacy.* Washington, DC: Author. Retrieved from https://health.gov/sites/default/files/2019-09/Health_Literacy_Action_Plan.pdf

U.S. Department of Health and Human Services, Office of Minority Health. (2016). *National standards for culturally and linguistically appropriate services in health and health care: Compendium of state-sponsored national CLAS standards implementation activities.* Washington, DC: Author.

Washington, K., Craig, K., Parker Oliver, D., Ruggeri, J., Brunk, S., & Goldstein, A. (2019). Family caregivers' perspectives on communication with cancer care providers. *Journal of Psychosocial Oncology, 37*(6), 777–790. https://doi.org/10.1080/07347332.2019.1624674

Wiles, J., Moeke-Maxwell, T., Williams, L., Black, S., Trussardi, G., & Gott, M. (2018). Caregivers for people at end of life in advanced age: Knowing, doing and negotiating care. *Age Ageing, 47*(6), 887–895. https://doi.org/10.1093/ageing/afy129

Wittenberg, E., Goldsmith, J., Ferrell, B., & Platt, C. S. (2015). Enhancing communication related to symptom management through plain language: A brief report. *Journal of Pain & Symptom Management, 50*(5), 707–711. https://doi.org/10.1016/j.jpainsymman.2015.06.007

Wittenberg, E., Goldsmith, J. V., Ragan, S., & Parnell, T. A. (2020). *Communication and palliative nursing: The COMFORT model* (2nd ed.). New York, NY: Oxford.

Wittenberg, E., Xu, J., Goldsmith, J., & Mendoza, Y. (2019). Caregiver communication about cancer: Development of a mhealth resource to support family caregiver communication burden. *Psychooncology, 28*(2), 365–371. https://doi.org/10.1002/pon.4950

Wittenberg-Lyles, E., Demiris, G., Parker Oliver, D., Washington, K., Burt, S., & Shaunfield, S. (2012). Stress variances among informal hospice caregivers. *Qualitative Health Research, 22*(8), 1114–1125. https://doi.org/10.1177/1049732312448543

Wolff, J. L., Guan, Y., Boyd, C. M., Vick, J., Amjad, H., Roth, D. L., . . . Roter, D. L. (2017). Examining the context and helpfulness of family companion contributions to older adults' primary care visits. *Patient Education & Counseling, 100*(3), 487–494. https://doi.org/10.1016/j.pec.2016.10.022

Wolters Kluwer Health: Lippincott Williams and Wilkins. (2015, October 15). Trained medical interpreters can reduce errors in care for patients with limited English proficiency. *Science Daily.* Retrieved from www.sciencedaily.com/releases/2015/10/151015132312.htm

World Health Organization. (2019). *About social determinants of health.* Retrieved from https://www.who.int/social_determinants/sdh_definition/en/

Yuen, E. Y., Knight, T., Dodson, S., Ricciardelli, L., Burney, S., & Livingston, P. M. (2014). Development of the health literacy of caregivers scale–Cancer (HLCS-C): Item generation and content validity testing. *BMC Family Practice, 15,* 202. https://doi.org/10.1186/s12875-014-0202-9

Zong, J., & Batalova, J. (2015, July 8). The Limited English proficient population in the United States. *Migration Information Source.* https://www.migrationpolicy.org/article/limited-english-proficient-population-united-states

3

Palliative Care

Paul, the home health nurse, called several times, suggesting talking to Dad about hospice. I could not do it. Dad still was fighting and as long as he wanted to fight, good for him! Mom and I talked about it [hospice]. I proceeded to attempt to learn all I could. I learned the difference between curative and palliative medicine. Finally, I decided to talk to Dad. My strength was gone but we knew we had to take the next steps. Dad sat in a recliner as we began to talk to him. I said, "Dad, I do not know how much longer Mom and I can take care of you. Maybe we need some help." My goodness it was hard to say. He agreed it was getting difficult. I suggested we could get help from hospice care. He thought and agreed. I went outside and called Paul (home health nurse). Paul came to see Dad. I was there when he got there. I asked Paul to talk to Dad about hospice. Paul explained what was possible. Dad listened intently to every word.

—Gary, son of cancer patient Von

The uncertainty of chronic illness, marked by a wide range of pain and other symptoms, disease flare-ups, or scan results showing reduction in disease leaves patients and caregivers with an unpredictable disease trajectory. When healthcare providers use ambivalent messages about disease, results, or the future, caregivers like Gary must rely on their own health literacy and communication skills to make decisions about care. System complexity, lack of available resources, provider time constraints, and fragmentation of services across the continuum of care contribute to the caregiver's navigation difficulties (Fields et al., 2018). As this opening quote depicts, these navigation difficulties are even more challenging when they involve communicating about transitions in care, especially when this transition involves hospice and palliative care. The nature of chronic disease demands a health-literate care organization to involve caregivers in the healthcare system and learn about the pre-existing structure and function of the family system. Caregiver communication patterns and needs require a tailored response from providers and the resources offered through systems. We describe *palliative care* in this chapter to illustrate how the patient and family's illness journey is powerfully influenced by their understanding of the disease and disease trajectory.

CAREGIVER INVOLVEMENT IN THE HEALTHCARE SYSTEM

> I will never forget the look on the "Prostate wives" faces as they stood outside the rooms in the "'Prostate wing." Feeling scared and alone, I sarcastically said to one woman, "Where is the support group session for partners being held? Oh, excuse me. There doesn't seem to be one." She responded with a sad look and said, "Yes, I know what you mean. Isn't that the truth?" We received thorough medical instructions regarding post-surgery issues, a list of resources, a few pages on sexual recovery, a list of both men and women, who would be willing to discuss their journeys with prostate cancer, and encouragement to call whenever we had any questions. I never felt comfortable calling a stranger on this list. I searched the web, contacted our local American Cancer Society and a prostate support group that I read about in our local newspaper. People were always kind to listen but there was little if any follow through in regard to my desire to become involved.
>
> —Mary, whose 49-year-old husband was diagnosed with prostate cancer

No one wants to be placed in a position where responsibilities are unclear, the magnitude of tasks is enormous and never-ending, little information is available to get help and support, and there are high expectations for success. Yet this is what is asked of caregivers! So much of their ability to be involved in a patient's healthcare depends on what they can find out about their tasks, where to get information, who to ask for help, when things should be done, and how to do things at home. Caregivers need to know about the patient's disease, understand why their help is needed and what their role is, learn about medication and treatment regimens, and be aware of the patient's wishes (Schulman-Green & Feder, 2018). This requires a healthcare system that formally defines and supports the family caregiver's active role in patient self-management.

Improvements to healthcare organizations, delivery systems, and health education are needed to provide support for patients who live with multiple chronic illnesses and are reliant on family caregiver involvement (Porter et al., 2019). The most popular approach for making system changes is the chronic care model (CCM), which has guided national quality improvement initiatives since its inception and is the foundation for most medical home models. It is a framework that provides organizations with a roadmap to identify general ideas for system-level changes that can be made to healthcare delivery practices and processes. The CCM identifies six interrelated system changes aimed at improving patient health outcomes through patient-centered, evidence-based care: healthcare organization; self-management support; delivery system design; decision support; clinical information; and community partners. Changes based on CCM implementation involve structural alteration to care practices and participation from nurses, physicians, social workers, patients, and caregivers.

While organizations that implement changes based on CCM improve quality of care and patient outcomes (Coleman et al., 2009), the model presents a linear approach to caring for each condition separately with each component individually generating favorable experiences (Boehmer et al., 2018). To date, no CCM implementation studies have been conducted on patients with multiple chronic conditions; meanwhile, the management of chronic illness remains complicated by multiple sources of information that are not integrated across healthcare systems or providers (Grover & Joshi, 2014). The formal integration of family caregivers into the care process is necessary to ensure that adequate information is provided about treatment options, treatment outcomes, consequences for caregivers' lives, hospital processes, and transitions back home (Preisler et al., 2019). And, importantly, this integration also must move beyond the provision of information; it must also offer care for the caregiver and attend to the specific day-to-day needs and priorities of this/these individual(s) and strive to tailor the responsiveness of stakeholders to caregiver needs.

Chronic illness care can be improved if delivery systems implement changes to include caregivers in all aspects of care. When caregivers are involved, patients have better care experiences, and both patient and caregiver experience better clinical outcomes (Wieczorek et al., 2018). We propose that inclusion of the caregiver is crucial to achieving proactive, structured, and planned care required to address multimorbidity among a growing patient population. The health-literate care model provides a framework for developing an organizational environment that encourages engagement of staff, patients, families, and caregivers and ultimately fosters care of the caregiver. The health literate care model incorporates principles of health literacy by embedding the Health Literacy Universal Precautions Toolkit within the six elements of the CCM (Koh et al., 2013). Table 3.1 provides a proposed overview of the health-literate care module that includes the family caregiver.

Expanding on ideas from CCM, the health-literate care model identifies ways to integrate caregivers into collaborative assessment, goal setting, action planning, and problem-solving patient goals (Koh et al., 2013). Most U.S. healthcare systems do not have an official platform for incorporating caregivers in the plan of care, and caregivers are not typically assessed to determine if they have any relevant knowledge for home-based care and support (Kent et al., 2016). For caregivers to be proactive in the patient's care (delivery system design), they need to be able to view the patient's medical records (clinical information systems) and have support in being able to understand the information they are viewing (decision support); caregivers also must be taught how to support patient care tasks at home (self-management support). Designed to strengthen the relationship between the healthcare team and patient, the health-literate care model offers a starting point for establishing processes to support caregiver communication and health

Table 3.1. Overview of the Health Literate Care Model Inclusive of the Family Caregiver

Health Literate Care Model Element[a]	Health Literate Care Model Example[a]	Health Literate Care Model Example with Caregivers
Healthcare organization *Establishing health-literate culture through leadership, planning, and operations*	• Quality improvement goals for addressing health literacy are set based on assessments and patient feedback with continuous monitoring of results • Systemwide training of workforce occurs in clear communication, health literacy universal precautions and skills	• Routine assessment of caregiver feedback via survey or other means • Quality improvement goals established based on caregiver feedback
Self-management support *Using strategies to promote self-management, check for understanding, and development of personal action plans*	• Teach-back method is used with every patient in every patient interaction • All self-management support resources follow principles of plain language and health literacy	• Team members are trained to include and address caregiver when delivering patient education • Personal action plan is developed for the caregiver that addresses needs for self-management support, caregiver health, and caregiver mental health
Delivery system design *Team-based care wherein team members have new roles and workflows*	• Brown bag medication review is routinely incorporated into the team's workflow • Team members follow up to verify patients' comprehension of care plans • Team members are proactive in arranging for language assistance services when needed	• A team member is designated to provide caregiver education • Team meetings/rounds include a report on the caregiver's understanding of the care plan, lab results, medications, and tests

(continued)

Table 3.1. CONTINUED

Health Literate Care Model Element[a]	Health Literate Care Model Example[a]	Health Literate Care Model Example with Caregivers
Decision support *Engage in shared decision-making (e.g., use of decision aids, culturally and linguistically appropriate materials)*	• The team provides self-paced, interactive patient decision aids • Providers engage in informed, shared decision-making conversations with patients with cultural humility	• Team members are trained to ask the patient about preferences for caregiver involvement • Caregiver information needs are assessed and addressed in a culturally and linguistically appropriate manner
Clinical information *Real-time reminders, access to view personal health record, online education*	• Teams receive reminders for health literacy-related tasks • Personal health records include patients' care plans, health-literate decision aids, self-management tools, and links to community resources and services	• Information systems include a caregiver portal • Electronic Medical Records include standardized caregiver health literacy information and learning preferences • Online education provided for caregivers in plain language
Community partners *Address needs based on social determinants of health and refer to community resources*	• The team develops referral relationships with providers of adult education and other essential nonmedical support • The team collaborates with community partners around health literacy universal precautions and culturally competent principles	• The team develops a contact list for local resources for home-based care and provides this to caregivers • One team member's job description includes maintaining relationships with community resources available to the caregiver

[a]From: Koh, H. K., Brach, C., Harris, L. M., & Parchman, M. L. (2013). A proposed "health literate care model" would constitute a systems approach to improving patients' engagement in care. *Health Affairs (Millwood)*, *32*(2), 357–367. doi:10.1377/hlthaff.2012.1205

literacy. With a focus on written and spoken communication, signage, e-health access, and the caregiver's access to these things, a health-literate health organization makes it easier for caregivers to navigate, understand, and use information to support patient self-management (Brach, 2017).

PALLIATIVE CARE AND FAMILY CAREGIVERS

A health-literate care organization is one that involves palliative care, an area of healthcare that recognizes family as central to the unit of care (National Consensus Project for Quality Palliative Care, 2018). According to the World Health Organization (2018), "Palliative Care is an approach that improves the quality of life of patients and their families facing the problems associated with life-threatening illness, through the prevention and relief of suffering by means of early identification and impeccable assessment and treatment of pain and other problems, physical, psychosocial and spiritual." Palliative care in the United States began in the 1990s as "comfort care," or care that could be offered to patients when curative care no longer worked. Initially practiced, palliative care was regarded as end-of-life care for late-stage, dying patients who no longer were being helped by medical efforts to treat or cure their diseases. Essentially, palliative care was tantamount to hospice care. Today, however, palliative care is very different from hospice care.

Hospice is a type of palliative care for people who have six months or less to live. It is provided to both the patient and family and includes attention to the physical, psychological, spiritual, and emotional needs of the dying. It is provided in many settings: home, nursing home, assisted living facility, or inpatient hospital. Although the U.S. Medicare Hospice Benefit affords terminally ill patients six months of hospice care, most patients use hospice care for fewer than 24 days (National Hospice and Palliative Care Organization, 2019). One reason why patients and families aren't using hospice for the full extent of their eligible benefits is because physicians must refer them to hospice and most providers have difficulty communicating about hospice or difficulty determining the best time to refer to hospice care (Hawley, 2017). When physicians are uncomfortable navigating end-of-life discussions and have a less positive attitude toward hospice, the result is more aggressive care and higher end-of-life spending (Keating et al., 2018).

Nationally, individuals with advanced disease are referred to hospice very late in their illness journey (Allsop et al., 2018), and most patients die receiving aggressive treatments (Mulville et al., 2019). Providers also refer too late to hospice because the course of disease is unpredictable in chronic illness, and chronic illness has not previously received palliative care support (Allsop et al., 2018). For example, providers have difficulty predicting death for individuals living with dementia (Armstrong et al., 2019), and a lack awareness of palliative care keeps them from addressing the topic with patient/family members (Erel et al., 2017). Similarly, patients on hemodialysis have less predictive illness trajectories and providers who are less willing to communicate about the prognostic outcomes of their patients resulting in very low hospice use, averaging six days (O'Hare et al., 2018).

In the absence of a health-literate delivery system, patient and family may receive conflicting messages from different specialty teams (e.g., between palliative care and oncology or between primary physician and palliative care; Newlin & Michener, 2019). Decision support is therefore not available to patient/family who then must choose between their specialty teams and sometimes between the team and their primary care physician. With multiple healthcare providers involved in chronic illness care, clinical information about referral to hospice may be miscommunicated among members of the healthcare team.

For good reason, there is a lack of hospice health literacy, with a misconception that hospice is only for care immediately before death. This results from a lack of trust, discomfort in talking about death (among providers/patients/family), and preference and reliance on religious beliefs over medical advice (Cicolello & Anandarajah, 2019). For example, among Latinos on hemodialysis, barriers to hospice care include family reluctance to have advance care planning discussions (Cervantes et al., 2017). However, when both patient and caregiver understand that the disease is incurable, they are more likely to prefer hospice (Trevino et al., 2019).

Today, the principles of hospice are applied to a broader population (including those with chronic illness) through palliative care, with the goal of reaching these patients much earlier in their illness or disease process (Casey, 2019). "Palliative care seeks to address physical pain and disease symptoms, along with emotional, social, and spiritual pain, to achieve the best possible quality of life for patients and their families" (Casey, 2019, p. 196). Palliative care permits patients to receive curative, life-prolonging treatment simultaneously with receiving care that enhances quality of life. It is holistic care that treats the whole person, not merely the disease. It involves both curative medical care by physicians, nurses, and other healthcare providers and also emotional, psychological, and spiritual care by a team of specialists including social workers, psychologists, and chaplains. While early literature in palliative care looked exclusively at end-of-life care, patients are now receiving the comforts of palliative care as they suffer chronic, not necessarily terminal, illnesses, making family caregivers even more central and critical to the caregiving process.

FAMILY CAREGIVER COMMUNICATION AND PALLIATIVE CARE

While palliative care services remain inconsistently installed across care settings and are not accessible to some patients and families, a *palliative care approach* to communication about chronic illness is needed to create awareness and understanding of disease and end-of-life trajectory for the patient and family. The diagnosis of a chronic illness marks a shift in the patient's story, redefining normal as "life before illness" and the future as "abnormal and damaged" (Porter et al., 2019). What is at stake in chronic illness is the family's ability to mobilize, come together, and communicate with each other to adapt to changes and execute the best care possible for the patient. We now share narratives about each caregiver's care recipient and the story of chronic illness that changes the course of life for each of our four caregivers.

Maggie Burkhart

Maggie's mom, Earlene, was the sole caregiver of her husband during his seven-month cancer journey. After his death, she settled into a new daily schedule of going to the store, visiting her doctors when she had appointments, and keeping up with the house. Her children visited intermittently from out of town, with the nearest daughter only 45 minutes away. During the next few years Earlene stuck closer and closer to the house and ventured out only once a week at most. One evening, Earlene phoned Maggie very upset about her remote control. Earlene felt as though it was a new remote that her kids had introduced into the home without telling Earlene, and she could not figure out how to use it. Maggie did her best to walk Earlene through the frustration but to no avail. When they spoke the next day, Earlene did not recall the trouble with the remote.

A month later, a neighbor of Earlene's called Maggie to report an incident with their mom. Earlene had asked the neighbor for help in turning off a light inside the car. The neighbor obliged and spent quite a bit of time with Earlene in her car looking for a light that was on. There was no light on. Earlene insisted that someone had been coming and turning a light on in her car, but she couldn't determine what light was on. Maggie's sisters elected to visit Earlene the following weekend. During their visit, Earlene came down with a virulent stomach virus and was so weakened that she needed their help for the next week. During this visit, her daughters discovered milk and eggs in the kitchen cabinets, spoiled food in the refrigerator, and bills that Earlene had paid multiple times.

Sharon Jenks

Sharon's partner Kelley felt strong and maintained her intense biking regimen until the summer. She was experiencing a recurring dull pain in her chest and described it as very generalized. Upon the urging of Sharon, they made a trip to the emergency room (ER) downtown, as they were preparing to leave in two days for a vacation trip out of state. A visit to the ER went from bad to worse as the diagnostics became increasingly complicated with bad news. Upon their discharge, she and her partner, Sharon, were told there was a very good likelihood that Kelley had lung cancer. While in the ER, she underwent a lung biopsy to positively identify the pathology in her lung. They had been warned of the levels of lethality that belonged to the various kinds of lung cancer. Mesothelioma was mentioned as the worst of the worst. She was doubtful of this diagnosis because she had never worked or lived near asbestos or other strong environmental indicators for the disease. She was a woman in her early 50s, much younger than the typical person who receives this diagnosis. Feeling hopeful that mesothelioma could not be the accurate diagnosis, but gripped with worry, she and Sharon ventured on to their long-awaited vacation.

While vacationing just days later, Kelley received a call from her internist announcing that the pathogen was cancer and that it was pleural mesothelioma. She embarked on a curative treatment process. Almost immediately, Kelley had to resign from her position as a media promoter to recover from the powerfully disabling effects of chemotherapy and radiation. First attempting two rounds of chemotherapy with moderate therapeutic effect, Kelley and Sharon opted to leave their primary oncologist and enter a trial at a neighboring cancer research center. Initial results were very positive, despite the frightening informed consent warnings and powerfully bad malaise. After two months of research protocol treatment, Kelley became dehydrated at home and nearly died. The couple was unable to receive service or attention from the research hospital and withdrew from the protocol. They returned to their previous oncology practice and were welcomed back.

Estella Rodriguez

Father to Estella, Marco Rodriguez fell during a daily walk in January. In his mid-70s, he was very active, able, and independent. He and his wife maintained their own home in South Texas and enjoyed their four children who all lived within three hours of them. Marco continued his regular daily activities while experiencing pain for a few days, went to his local physician, and received a clean bill of health. By July, Marco was still complaining of pain and became incapacitated while working in the yard. A general practitioner saw Marco and referred him to a "cancer doctor." He proceeded on to an oncologist, not understanding he had been diagnosed with advanced cancer, and instead describing his problem as a "hole in my leg." The family is still troubled about the method by which they learned about the seriousness of Marco's illness.

In an appointment with Marco's oncologist, the family learned that he was suffering from advanced stage multiple myeloma. At this late stage of illness, Marco's vertebrae and ribs were breaking even during minimal movement. His pain level soared, and by the fall, Marco was incapacitated and bed-ridden. His sons provided all of the day-to-day care for their parents. The family became frustrated with the oncologist as Marco's pain was never addressed, and they felt they were not taken seriously on this matter. In the midst of his excruciating pain, he underwent intensive chemotherapy treatments that were far more aggressive in their side effects than the family knew they would be; Marco lost 50 pounds in the course of a few months. By winter, Marco had deteriorated substantially and his pain curtailed any quality of life.

Viv Gray

Jake's symptoms for Gulf War illness probably had begun over two decades ago with rashes, irritable bowel, neuropathy, malaise, muscle pain, and confusion. His chronic pain and fatigue took shape after his deployment to Iraq in 1991. He was one of the youngest people in the military ever diagnosed with gout at the age of 21. This was followed by injuries in training, including broken tibias and torn ligaments. But his combat experience in the Middle East was the creator of his posttraumatic stress disorder (PTSD). Regular nighttime patrols, tactical intelligence gathering at night in dugout bunkers, and months of artillery fire took their toll and continue to. Trauma and anxiety had altered his processing and mental health. Fifteen years of addictions were an ineffective cover for his now-brittle PTSD. Once those addictions were removed, his pursuit of healthcare started in earnest, as did his precipitous decline in health.

A few months ago, a complete blood count test revealed high blood sugar that was confirmed via a glucose tolerance test. He now also carries the diagnosis of type 2 diabetes. On disability at the age of 50, Jake chases care and relief for several chronic conditions using the Veterans Administration benefit.

In his 20s and 30s, he was married and had four children. Once sober, the marriage did not survive. His family moved far away from him, and he struggled to find purpose at the same time he sought medical care for highly complex chronic illnesses. His own family (mom and sister) was very separate from him and operated independently. His dad died when Jake was a teenager. The re-entry of Viv in his life two decades after they were in high school brought clarity and direction to Jake's Veterans Affairs care. Viv worked every day to address at least one of the ongoing difficulties.

Jake had gained 50 pounds in the last six months. With each weigh in, his blood work told the sad story of worsening type 2 diabetes. Viv sought help from an endocrinologist and battled with his primary physician to get help with his polypharmacy, unresolved symptoms of neuropathy, and PTSD. The healthcare system was their biggest barrier. Gaining access to a specialist took between six and eight months. One particular challenge of this behavioral illness was Jake's inability to sleep at all at night. Once asleep, he would engage in a typical habit of those suffering with PTSD, eating while sleeping, worsening his type 2 diabetes.

These stories reflect elements of the symptoms, diagnosis, care navigation, and family contexts in chronic illness. Current healthcare organization practices place little emphasis on patient and family understanding; instead, emphasis is placed on giving information by holding a family meeting, sharing illness updates (e.g., test results, treatment options), or advance care planning. Healthcare team members are unclear about whose role it is to speak to the patient and family about end-of-life care, and many are uncomfortable talking about it (Thurston et al., 2016). As a result, disease trajectory is rarely integrated into discussions, especially the subject of end-of-life care. For example, patients with lung cancer and their family members reported little or no recall of physicians initiating discussions about concerns or an opportunity to engage in advance care planning and, additionally, reported a sense of abandonment upon facing end of life without the accompaniment of or conversation with their primary providers (Horne et al., 2019).

When patient and family lack understanding about the disease and disease trajectory, they are more likely to adopt a "do everything" approach to care. A "do everything" perspective from the family can occur when (a) the patient goes along with what family wants, (b) the patient is young (especially pediatric patient populations), or (c) the patient or family actually do want everything to be done. This "do everything" term must be teased out by providers with patient and family as it can also include a focus on comfort care, such as palliative care (Hopeck, 2018). During chronic illness, patients' and families' learning needs span the continuum of care (Christensen, 2017). A person's ability to process information and retain it is affected by the setting in which information is exchanged. Families who are able to openly talk about the disease are better able to support patients' preferences for care, navigate the practical demands of care, and come to terms with difficult issues (Foster et al., 2015). This volume offers the opportunity to consider other family communication patterns and resulting caregiver burdens—when families are unable to openly talk about disease or support a patient's preferences.

FAMILY COMMUNICATION AND THE NATURE OF CHRONIC DISEASE

There are a number of disease factors that give shape to the way that families talk about and organize themselves to care for a family member with a chronic illness (Rolland, 2018). These factors have been identified by Rolland (2018) as the family illness systems model. First, the *onset of disease* as either an acute crisis or gradual onset influences the mobilization of family and family adaptation. In an acute crisis, family communication is heightened and prioritized to bring family together. Families are sometimes able to come together on their own, allowing providers to focus on aiding family decision-making and mediating family relationships. The gradual onset of chronic illness, such as Alzheimer's disease, can create a less clear cause to rally for family to understand and communicate about the disease.

The family's ability to adapt and change roles within the family also depends upon the *course of disease*. Diseases such as Alzheimer's disease and chronic obstructive pulmonary disease often have a *progressive* disease course with continual symptoms followed by a gradual decline. Caregiving tasks emerge as the disease progresses, creating the need for ongoing adjustment. Vital to this disease course is family adaptability, as disease progression requires changes to the family's home and family organization (Whitehead et al., 2018). Figuring out how to integrate illness into family life and make necessary adjustments takes place over time (Robinson, 2017). Whether or not responsibilities for care are shared among family members or faced by one caregiver alone, increasing strain is felt by the family due to long disease duration and slow progression. A *relapsing/episodic* disease course, which can occur commonly in type 2 diabetes and multiple sclerosis, alternates between stable periods of varying length with low symptoms and "flare ups" in which symptoms are exacerbated.

Cancer survivorship, on the other hand, has a *constant* chronic disease course in which there is an event (diagnosis) and then stabilization (remission). As a result of long-term and late effects of cancer treatment, cancer survivors are likely to have multiple chronic conditions (Guy et al., 2017; Jacobs & Shulman, 2017). Cancer caregivers are often thrust into the role which emerges at diagnosis. Unlike other chronic illnesses such as dementia, cancer can bring rapid patient decline in a short period of time causing caregivers to provide more intense care over a brief period. Cancer disease onset may be sudden, with no major symptoms or family history, and lingering concerns about recurrence can remain, creating a state of ongoing caregiving (Rolland, 2005). Patient pain and the scope of the caregiver's pain management responsibilities also vary due to multimodal therapies, requiring caregivers to monitor symptoms more frequently and to address psychosocial aspects of health promotion during treatment.

The anticipated *outcome of the disease* also influences the family's willingness to discuss end-of-life care, and different end-of-life trajectories impact anticipatory grieving (Coelho et al., 2018). The family's perception and understanding about whether or not the disease will cause death or shorten the lifespan impacts how they approach advanced care planning and discuss end-of-life care. However, prognostic uncertainty is common in chronic illness, and most healthcare providers are unable to guide families into timely end-of-life care discussions (Krawczyk & Gallagher, 2016). With little guidance about the outcome of the disease from providers, end-of-life communication is often stymied within the family, and family members may engage in overprotection and concealment by not talking about the disease. For example, some families choose not to discuss a cancer diagnosis, as they have difficulty accepting the prognosis and difficulty coping, not wanting to upset others, and not knowing what to say (Bowen et al., 2017). Similarly, some family members choose not to disclose or discuss the diagnosis with the person who has dementia (van Wijngaarden et al., 2018).

Finally, the degree to which the patient is *incapacitated* deeply affects family coping and stress. Depending on the illness, patient decline can occur incrementally, with family members problem-solving and adjusting as the disease progresses or all at once at the time of diagnosis or an acute event. The extent, kind, and type of decline varies, and social stigma from disease class (HIV/AIDS, hepatitis) and/or disfigurement can contribute to family stress. In dementia, for example, cognitive decline creates aggression, agitation, and repetitive speech; caregivers report that this challenging behavior contributes to caregiver fatigue and stress (Slaboda et al., 2018). Given that the psychosocial factors of illness impact family stress and coping, adaptability, mobilization, and functioning, an integrated palliative care approach is necessary to improve chronic illness care.

ILLNESS JOURNEYS

A palliative care approach addresses the unique needs of family caregivers within the healthcare system and focuses on the importance of communication among patient, family caregivers, and healthcare providers. The involvement of palliative care services and willingness to discuss palliative care topics is highly dependent upon how palliative care is introduced and whether or not the family caregiver understands palliative care. Caregivers for the chronically ill are painfully unaware of palliative care and among those who have heard of palliative care, the majority do not see it as separate from hospice care and death (Dionne-Odom et al., 2019). Racial minorities (non-Whites) and those without a college degree are less likely to know about palliative care (Dionne-Odom et al., 2019).

When there is no designated role for the family caregiver within the healthcare delivery system, caregivers use past personal healthcare experiences (e.g., their own healthcare or prior caregiving experience) as well as prior deaths of other family members to guide their communication and decision-making (Moss et al., 2019). Family members often have difficulty accepting prognoses and can go against the patient's wishes and advance directives when the patient is incapacitated (Beckstrand et al., 2018). The strain of their caregiving roles makes family caregivers particularly in need of specialized palliative and hospice care support, yet their ignorance sorely reduces their chances of receiving such support.

Facilitating palliative care and being responsible for the continuity of care exacts strong health literacy and patient/family centered care in chronic illness (Reigada et al., 2015). Not having palliative care explained adequately and suboptimal provider–patient–caregiver communication are barriers to achieving the most effective approach to complex chronic illness (Boucher et al., 2018). There are three entry points by which patients and families either do or do not encounter palliative care when they are faced with chronic illness: the *isolated journey* for which palliative care does not exist; the *rescued journey* for which palliative care happens late in the disease course; and the *comforted journey* for which palliative care occurs early in the illness and is present throughout (Wittenberg-Lyles et al., 2011).

ISOLATED JOURNEY

When the family and patient are not openly aware of the need to adapt and adjust to chronic illness and its potential comorbidities, they experience the *isolated journey*. The isolated journey never has a turning point toward quality of life. Instead, the focus remains on restoring the patient's body to "normal." A variety of specialists and interdisciplinary providers are involved, but they lack knowledge about palliative care and the communication skills needed to introduce the topic to patient and family. There is no clinical information structure to facilitate development of a unified plan of care for the patient or to alert providers for necessary testing or the need for palliative care. Healthcare team members may meet with patient and family; however, communication barriers are common, including the lack of availability of a private setting, interruptions from staff, and scheduling occurring at the convenience of the providers, which restricts family attendance. Patient and family participation in meetings is often limited due to a lack of trust or a top–down approach to communication, which impedes patient decision-making support. Caregivers are left scrambling to learn and navigate multiple healthcare systems. There is a continued search for medical care and therapies despite the reality of the patient's chronic illness. At this point patients and their families can misunderstand that the disease is chronic, and despite a diagnosis, they perceive that little change in the practices of daily living is needed.

A lack of health literate communication creates enormous disillusionment and confusion for patients and families in this journey. They circuitously search for their disease path and for drugs and methods to tame the course; they often experience anger with providers for not being more vigilant as their disease process intensifies. Family and patient energy is channeled into treatment-focused, active care. Time and opportunity to live less sickly and solve more personal and family problems are lost in this journey. Suppressed discussions about future needs serve to further abuse family and patient when decline ensues. There is no preparation for decline and complications in chronic illness. There is no plan for future end-of-life care. There has been little or no discussion about illness trajectories, patient wishes, or place of care. The family and patient navigate this journey alone; when the patient can no longer participate in the journey due to delirium, pain, or unconsciousness, unanswered questions surrounding decision-making, responsibility, problem-solving, fear, and isolation can further traumatize a family.

In a healthcare organization that is not health literate, an isolated journey is more likely to occur. Throughout this journey, there is a lack of community, aid, or answers, and limited knowledge of available community resources that could improve engagement and the care experience. There is an absence of self-management support tools; staff and providers have not been adequately trained in health literacy support; and there is a lack of knowledge regarding teaching methods that check for understanding and track patient and caregiver goals. Caregivers are left feeling unprepared, in chaos, standing alone, without support or protection, and detached from the healthcare setting and system. When caregivers face health literacy related barriers such as difficulty communicating and navigating for services and support, patients suffer a decline in mental health and physical outcomes and experience more unmet needs (Sklenarova et al., 2015).

RESCUED JOURNEY

A plethora of treatment choices and options are offered for individuals with chronic illness with the presumption that active care displaces death and dying as a distant, deniable possibility. When patient preferences are not discussed, open communication about course of disease is missing, and patient/family understanding are not considered; the focus of care remains on treatment and leaves the patient and family careening toward a chaotic period of escalating interventions (Dillworth et al., 2016). At some point, however, the patient declines from either progressive disease or as a result of multiple chronic conditions, and end-of-life care is needed. When healthcare providers talk openly about disease and expectations for remaining length of life, patient and family are more likely to choose comfort over treatment; more often than not, they choose hospice (Gramling et al., 2019). Palliative care limited to hospice requires patient/family understanding about the course of disease and depicts the rescued journey experienced by the majority of Americans today.

The rescue confronts patients and their families who have experienced prolonged suffering, treatments, and numerous visits with independent healthcare providers with no real understanding of the magnitude or course of the disease. When a family is exposed to hospice when the patient is actively dying, this increases the difficulty for families to accept death and dying as part of their loved one's illness journey, making the move to and care in hospice a frustrating experience (Dalal & Bruera, 2017). This also reduces the time for necessary discussions about end-of-life care issues, leaving patients and family members with a limited understanding of end-of-life care. When family is insufficiently prepared for the patient's death, conflict emerges as an emotion, which triggers concerns about care (Francois et al., 2017). The lack of information and time in hospice care results in a turbulent dislocation of patients and family members despite their move from the isolated to the rescued journey.

Families experiencing the rescued journey are common in our healthcare system today. In 2019, it was estimated that one in every three deaths in the United States was under hospice care (National Hospice and Palliative Care Organization, 2019). These patients and families aggressively sought a variety of therapies for multiple chronic conditions. Similar to isolated patients and families, the energy of this group is also channeled into finding, receiving, and recovering from therapies despite the cost of time and futility (Allsop et al., 2018). This population has little understanding of the diseases they are facing and little exposure to hospice and palliative care in the course of illness. Patient and family are rescued from an isolated journey when they gain knowledge and understanding of the patient's condition right at the end of life.

This journey, although we frame it as a rescue, is wrought with conflict and difficult realities for a family. After months or years of focusing on active care, transition to comfort care in a matter of moments can be most difficult and impossible to accept. Some patients and families harbor intense resentment toward their primary physician(s) or the hospice team—as they can be seen as the bearers of unexpected news. Some families experience hospice as a brutal stage in comprehending their loved one's illness journey. These families remain isolated within the resources of hospice care as they continue to set expectations that are conducive with survival rather than comfort. Since patients and families have been offered a myriad of interventional treatment choices, a transition to hospice care negates this interventional behavior and introduces what many patients and families consider a passive role in the care process. Families struggle with the guilt of hospice placement as a result of misunderstanding the prognosis and disease trajectory, and a short time with hospice impedes them from relocating their loved one's illness journey as one that includes end of life. All of these reasons point to the need for a change in our healthcare system to a health-literate care organization that shifts the focus from merely communicating to promoting patient and family understanding, supporting shared decision making and fostering engagement. As described in the following section the comforted journey is embedded in a health literate care organization guided by early palliative care.

COMFORTED JOURNEY

Patients and families in the comforted journey receive both chronic illness care and palliative care. The presence of palliative care throughout the disease trajectory ensures far more thorough attention to and protection from suffering for a patient and family. An awareness of serious illness is integrated into initial and subsequent discussions about prognosis and care choices. This heavily impacts shared goals that patients and their physicians plan and execute, reducing the disillusionment that dominates treatment and care for patients with chronic illness. The comforted journey is delivered by the interdisciplinary palliative care team that includes physicians, nurses, social workers, chaplains, psychologists, and potentially other team members who could offer support. These differing roles are put into place for the holistic care of the patient and family so that the many aspects of psychosocial transition can be addressed as identities shift and care plans are established. The interdisciplinary team is constructed essentially to represent, support, and comfort patients/families as they face the most difficult care decisions and the stress of caregiving.

Caregivers present themselves to healthcare providers in a variety of ways, sometimes as highly health literate and with more than adequate family support. So how can you tell when a caregiver is struggling with caregiving? Palliative care offers a comprehensive set of clinical practice guidelines for attending to the needs of family caregivers. These guidelines specify the domains of palliative care as shown in Figure 3.1 and detail the many ways that providers can learn about the family structure that reveal communication patterns of caregivers.

Palliative care promotes (a) shared goals among all healthcare providers and their units of care—the patient and family—and (b) the reduction of suffering for all. This goal is simply nonexistent in the isolated journey and is not engaged until the end of the rescued journey. The comforted journey provides a community of professionals who make the experience of the patient/family their primary concern and transitions patients/families through stages of care. In the comforted journey, health literacy is integrated throughout palliative care and chronic illness.

Healthcare organizations can emphasize a health-literate culture by establishing palliative care leadership, planning for palliative care education that incorporates health literacy, and installing operations and policy that support interprofessional team practice to enable whole person care that includes the caregiver. The

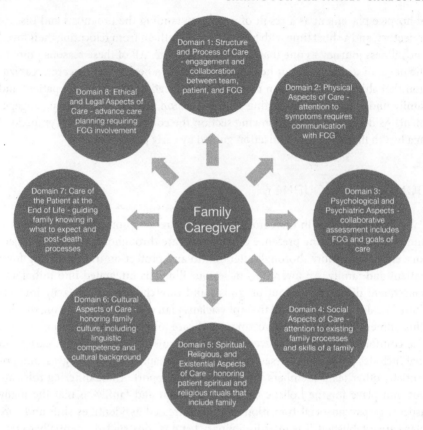

Figure 3.1. The family caregiver as central to national consensus project domains of palliative care.
NOTE: FCG = family caregiver.
SOURCE: National Consensus Project for Quality Palliative Care. (2018). *Clinical practice guidelines for quality palliative care*. Retrieved from https://www.nationalcoalitionhpc. org/ncp.

inclusion of palliative care within the system adds to the likelihood that *clinical information systems* will include "triggers" for palliative care referral for individuals with chronic illness. The system alerts providers to the patient/family need for palliative care and enables communication between specialty services. The interprofessional landscape of palliative care ensures that *community partners* are utilized as resources as palliative care social workers and chaplains assess social determinants of health and provide information about community resources. The *delivery system design* of palliative care affords team-based care wherein team members have new roles. *Decision support* includes use of decision aids and culturally and linguistically appropriate materials, and this is emphasized in clinical practice guidelines. National guidelines should be embedded into daily practice. *Self-management support* is enabled in palliative care as teams establish plans of care and mutual goal setting with patient/family. Palliative care emphasizes patient/family's role in managing health, skill development, and the development of personalized action plans.

A palliative care approach benefits family caregivers by including and involving them in patient care. As a result, palliative care achieves the "quadruple aim of healthcare": it improves patients' health; it improves patients' quality of life; it reduces unnecessary medical interventions, hospitalizations, and their associated costs; and it improves the work life of healthcare providers, clinicians, and staff (Bodenheimer & Sinsky, 2014). We also believe that inclusion of the family caregiver fosters enhanced health literacy, reducing caregiver communication burden and positively impacting caregiver outcomes. Moreover, "family caregiver awareness and perceptions of palliative care may help increase acceptance and access to timely palliative care by patients" (Bodenheimer & Sinsky, 2014, p. 6). This care may be particularly crucial to African American and other racial minorities and those with less education who receive aggressive curative treatments and intensive hospital-based care at end of life.

Morris (2015) reiterates that support for family caregivers and awareness of palliative care services are particularly relevant as chronically ill patients face end of life. The ideal situation is for caregivers to work in partnership with healthcare professionals to plan patient care and help manage their illness—yet the support needs of caregivers must also be addressed by healthcare providers (Morris et al., 2015). Whereas the caregiver role can be costly in terms of caregivers neglecting their own health and also suffering psychological distress, it can also reap the rewards of enhanced self-esteem, social approval, and the satisfaction of fulfilling a moral duty. Support needs of caregivers include psychological/emotional support; information; help with personal, nursing, and medical care of the patient; respite, and financial help (Morris et al., 2015).

CONCLUSION

Caring for an individual with multiple chronic conditions increases the caregiver's role; as care is more demanding, there is additional administrative and financial complexity, and additional coordination and communication needed among multiple healthcare providers (Boehmer et al., 2018). Caregivers facilitate communication with the patient (e.g., repeating information, asking questions, translating what was said during appointments) and communicate with the caregiving network (other family members, friends, community resources) and the healthcare team (Schaffler et al., 2019). As discussed in Chapter 1 of this volume, caregivers are often the bridge to all three parties, serving as intermediaries to the entire care process. They need to be knowledgeable about patient care and have the skills to describe care strategies, to express an opinion about care and request explanations of care, and redirect conversations with healthcare team members toward the patient (Dingley et al., 2017).

Implementing a health literate care model by fostering caregiver health literacy establishes formal integration and engagement of caregivers in the healthcare system. The three illness journeys described in this chapter illustrate the need to focus on communication with family caregivers and to build health literate organizations that include family caregivers as an essential component to chronic illness care. These journeys are presented to illustrate how health-literate healthcare organizations can engage, communicate with, and support family caregivers; enhance shared decision-making; and improve chronic disease management. "Palliative care has become the preeminent medical ally for anyone who wants to live a good life while coping with a debilitating illness" (Butler, 2019, p. 91). Palliative care communication with patient and family become essential in delivering quality care and helping patient and family to engage in open communication about chronic disease, life changes, and medical decisions.

REFERENCES

Allsop, M. J., Ziegler, L. E., Mulvey, M. R., Russell, S., Taylor, R., & Bennett, M. I. (2018). Duration and determinants of hospice-based specialist palliative care: A national retrospective cohort study. *Palliative Medicine, 32*(8), 1322–1333. https://doi.org/10.1177/0269216318781417

Armstrong, M. J., Alliance, S., Taylor, A., Corsentino, P., & Galvin, J. E. (2019). End-of-life experiences in dementia with Lewy bodies: Qualitative interviews with former caregivers. *PLoS One, 14*(5), e0217039. https://doi.org/10.1371/journal.pone.0217039

Beckstrand, R. L., Mallory, C., Macintosh, J. L. B., & Luthy, K. E. (2018). Critical care nurses' qualitative reports of experiences with family behaviors as obstacles in end-of-life care. *Dimension of Critical Care Nursing, 37*(5), 251–258. https://doi.org/10.1097/DCC.0000000000000310

Bodenheimer, T., & Sinsky, C. (2014). From triple to quadruple aim: Care of the patient requires care of the provider. *Annals of Family Medicine, 12*(6), 573–576. https://doi.org/10.1370/afm.1713

Boehmer, K. R., Abu Dabrh, A. M., Gionfriddo, M. R., Erwin, P., & Montori, V. M. (2018). Does the chronic care model meet the emerging needs of people living with multimorbidity? A systematic review and thematic synthesis. *PLoS One, 13*(2), e0190852. https://doi.org/10.1371/journal.pone.0190852

Boucher, N. A., Bull, J. H., Cross, S. H., Kirby, C., Davis, J. K., & Taylor, D. H., Jr. (2018). Patient, caregiver, and taxpayer knowledge of palliative care and views on a model of community-based palliative care. *Journal of Pain & Symptom Management, 56*(6), 951–956. https://doi.org/10.1016/j.jpainsymman.2018.08.007

Bowen, D. J., Hay, J. L., Harris-Wai, J. N., Meischke, H., & Burke, W. (2017). All in the family? Communication of cancer survivors with their families. *Familial Cancer, 16*(4), 597–603. https://doi.org/10.1007/s10689-017-9987-8

Brach, C. (2017). The journey to become a health literate organization: A snapshot of health system improvement. *Studies in Health Technology and Informatics, 240*, 203–237. https://www.ncbi.nlm.nih.gov/pubmed/28972519

Butler, K. (2019). *The art of dying well: A practical guide to a good end of life.* New York, NY: Simon & Schuster.

Casey, D. (2019). Hospice and palliative care: What's the difference? *Medsurg Nursing*, *28*(3), 196–197.

Cervantes, L., Jones, J., Linas, S., & Fischer, S. (2017). Qualitative interviews exploring palliative care perspectives of Latinos on dialysis. *Clinical Journal of the American Society of Nephrology*, *12*(5), 788–798. https://doi.org/10.2215/CJN.10260916

Christensen, D. (2017). The impact of health literacy on palliative care outcomes. *Journal of Hospice & Palliative Nursing*, *18*(6), 544–549.

Cicolello, K., & Anandarajah, G. (2019). Multiple stakeholders' perspectives regarding barriers to hospice enrollment in diverse patient populations: A qualitative study. *Journal of Pain & Symptom Management*, *57*(5), 869–879. https://doi.org/10.1016/j.jpainsymman.2019.02.012

Coelho, A., de Brito, M., & Barbosa, A. (2018). Caregiver anticipatory grief: Phenomenology, assessment and clinical interventions. *Current Opinion in Supportive Palliative Care*, *12*(1), 52–57. https://doi.org/10.1097/SPC.0000000000000321

Coleman, K., Austin, B. T., Brach, C., & Wagner, E. H. (2009). Evidence on the chronic care model in the new millennium. *Health Affairs (Millwood)*, *28*(1), 75–85. https://doi.org/10.1377/hlthaff.28.1.75

Dalal, S., & Bruera, E. (2017). End-of-life care matters: Palliative cancer care results in better care and lower costs. *Oncologist*, *22*(4), 361–368. https://doi.org/10.1634/theoncologist.2016-0277

Dillworth, J., Dickson, V. V., Mueller, A., Shuluk, J., Yoon, H. W., & Capezuti, E. (2016). Nurses' perspectives: Hospitalized older patients and end-of-life decision-making. *Nursing in Critical Care*, *21*(2), e1–e11. https://doi.org/10.1111/nicc.12125

Dingley, C. E., Clayton, M., Lai, D., Doyon, K., Reblin, M., & Ellington, L. (2017). Caregiver activation and home hospice nurse communication in advanced cancer care. *Cancer Nursing*, *40*(5), E38–E50. https://doi.org/10.1097/NCC.0000000000000429

Dionne-Odom, J. N., Ornstein, K. A., & Kent, E. E. (2019). What do family caregivers know about palliative care? Results from a national survey. *Palliative & Supportive Care*, *17*(6), 643–649. https://doi.org/10.1017/S1478951519000154

Erel, M., Marcus, E. L., & Dekeyser-Ganz, F. (2017). Barriers to palliative care for advanced dementia: A scoping review. *Annals of Palliative Medicine*, *6*(4), 365–379. https://doi.org/10.21037/apm.2017.06.13

Fields, B., Rodakowski, J., James, A. E., & Beach, S. (2018). Caregiver health literacy predicting healthcare communication and system navigation difficulty. *Families, Systems, & Health*, *36*(4), 482–492. https://doi.org/10.1037/fsh0000368

Foster, C., Myall, M., Scott, I., Sayers, M., Brindle, L., Cotterell, P., . . . Robinson, J. (2015). 'You can't say, "What about me?" I'm not the one with cancer': Information and support needs of relatives. *Psycho-Oncology*, *24*(6), 705–711. https://doi.org/10.1002/pon.3716

Francois, K., Lobb, E., Barclay, S., & Forbat, L. (2017). The nature of conflict in palliative care: A qualitative exploration of the experiences of staff and family members. *Patient and Education Counseling*, *100*(8), 1459–1465. https://doi.org/10.1016/j.pec.2017.02.019

Gramling, R., Ingersoll, L. T., Anderson, W., Priest, J., Berns, S., Cheung, K., . . . Alexander, S. C. (2019). End-of-life preferences, length-of-life conversations, and hospice enrollment in palliative care: A direct observation cohort study among people with advanced cancer. *Journal of Palliative Medicine, 22*(2), 152–156. https://doi.org/10.1089/jpm.2018.0476

Grover, A., & Joshi, A. (2014). An overview of chronic disease models: A systematic literature review. *Global Journal of Health Science, 7*(2), 210–227. https://doi.org/10.5539/gjhs.v7n2p210

Guy, G. P., Jr., Yabroff, K. R., Ekwueme, D. U., Rim, S. H., Li, R., & Richardson, L. C. (2017). Economic burden of chronic conditions among survivors of cancer in the United States. *Journal of Clinical Oncology, 35*(18), 2053–2061. https://doi.org/10.1200/JCO.2016.71.9716

Hawley, P. (2017). Barriers to access to palliative care. *Palliative Care, 10.* https://doi.org/10.1177/1178224216688887

Hopeck, P. (2018). Care providers' integration of family requests in end-of-life communication: Understanding what to do and why to do it. *Health Communication, 33*(10), 1277–1283. https://doi.org/10.1080/10410236.2017.1351273

Horne, G., Payne, S., & Seymour, J. (2019). Do patients with lung cancer recall physician-initiated discussions about planning for end-of-life care following disclosure of a terminal prognosis? *BMJ Supportive & Palliative Care, 9*(2), 197–201. https://doi.org/10.1136/bmjspcare-2015-001015

Jacobs, L. A., & Shulman, L. N. (2017). Follow-up care of cancer survivors: Challenges and solutions. *Lancet Oncology, 18*(1), e19–e29. https://doi.org/10.1016/S1470-2045(16)30386-2

Keating, N. L., Huskamp, H. A., Kouri, E., Schrag, D., Hornbrook, M. C., Haggstrom, D. A., & Landrum, M. B. (2018). Factors contributing to geographic variation in end-of-life expenditures for cancer patients. *Health Affairs (Millwood), 37*(7), 1136–1143. https://doi.org/10.1377/hlthaff.2018.0015

Kent, E. E., Rowland, J. H., Northouse, L., Litzelman, K., Chou, W. S., Shelburne, N., . . . Huss, K. (2016). Caring for caregivers and patients: Research and clinical priorities for informal cancer caregiving. *Cancer, 122*(13), 1987–1995. https://doi.org/10.1002/cncr.29939

Koh, H. K., Brach, C., Harris, L. M., & Parchman, M. L. (2013). A proposed "health literate care model" would constitute a systems approach to improving patients' engagement in care. *Health Affairs (Millwood), 32*(2), 357–367. https://doi.org/10.1377/hlthaff.2012.1205

Krawczyk, M., & Gallagher, R. (2016). Communicating prognostic uncertainty in potential end-of-life contexts: Experiences of family members. *BMC Palliative Care, 15,* 59. https://doi.org/10.1186/s12904-016-0133-4

Morris, S. M., King, C., Turner, M., & Payne, S. (2015). Family carers providing support to a person dying in the home setting: A narrative literature review. *Palliative Medicine, 29*(6), 487–495. https://doi.org/10.1177/0269216314565706

Moss, K. O., Douglas, S. L., Baum, E., & Daly, B. (2019). Family surrogate decision-making in chronic critical illness: A qualitative analysis. *Critical Care Nurse, 39*(3), e18–e26. https://doi.org/10.4037/ccn2019176

Mulville, A. K., Widick, N. N., & Makani, N. S. (2019). Timely referral to hospice care for oncology patients: A retrospective review. *American Journal of Hospice and Palliative Care, 36*(6), 466–471. https://doi.org/10.1177/1049909118820494

National Consensus Project for Quality Palliative Care. (2018). *Clinical practice guidelines for quality palliative care.* https://www.nationalcoalitionhpc.org/ncp

National Hospice and Palliative Care Organization. (2019). *Facts & figures: Hospice care in America*. Retrieved from http://www.nhpco.org

Newlin, E., & Michener, C. (2019). Barriers to hospice referral and opinions regarding the primary role of palliative care in gynecologic oncology. *Consult QD*. Retrieved from https://consultqd.clevelandclinic.org/barriers-to-hospice-referral-and-opinions-regarding-the-primary-role-of-palliative-care-in-gynecologic-oncology/

O'Hare, A. M., Hailpern, S. M., Wachterman, M., Kreuter, W., Katz, R., Hall, Y. N., . . . Daratha, K. B. (2018). Hospice use and end-of-life spending trajectories in medicare beneficiaries on hemodialysis. *Health Affairs (Millwood)*, *37*(6), 980–987. https://doi.org/10.1377/hlthaff.2017.1181

Porter, T., Ong, B. N., & Sanders, T. (2019). Living with multimorbidity? The lived experience of multiple chronic conditions in later life. *Health (London)*. https://doi.org/10.1177/1363459319834997

Preisler, M., Rohrmoser, A., Goerling, U., Kendel, F., Bar, K., Reimer, M., . . . Letsch, A. (2019). Early palliative care for those who care: A qualitative exploration of cancer caregivers' information needs during hospital stays. *European Journal of Cancer Care*, *28*(2), e12990. https://doi.org/https://doi.org/10.1111/ecc.12990

Reigada, C., Pais-Ribeiro, J., Novellas, A., & Gonçalves, E. (2015). The caregiver role in palliative care: A systematic review of the literature. *Health Care Current Reviews*, *3*(2), 143. https://doi.org/10.4172/2375-4273.1000143

Robinson, C. A. (2017). Families living well with chronic illness: The healing process of moving on. *Qualitative Health Research*, *27*(4), 447–461. https://doi.org/10.1177/1049732316675590

Rolland, J. S. (2005). Cancer and the family: An integrative model. *Cancer*, *104*(11 Suppl), 2584–2595. https://doi.org/10.1002/cncr.21489

Rolland, J. S. (2018). *Helping couples and families navigate illness and disability: An integrated approach*. New York, NY: Guilford Press.

Schaffler, J. L., Tremblay, S., Laizner, A. M., & Lambert, S. (2019). Developing education materials for caregivers of culturally and linguistically diverse patients: Insights from a qualitative analysis of caregivers' needs, access and understanding of information. *Health Expectations*, *22*(3), 444–456. https://doi.org/10.1111/hex.12867

Schulman-Green, D., & Feder, S. (2018). Integrating family caregivers into palliative oncology care using the self- and family management approach. *Seminars in Oncology Nursing*, *34*(3), 252–263. https://doi.org/10.1016/j.soncn.2018.06.006

Sklenarova, H., Krumpelmann, A., Haun, M. W., Friederich, H. C., Huber, J., Thomas, M., . . . Hartmann, M. (2015). When do we need to care about the caregiver? Supportive care needs, anxiety, and depression among informal caregivers of patients with cancer and cancer survivors. *Cancer*, *121*(9), 1513–1519. https://doi.org/10.1002/cncr.29223

Slaboda, J., Fail, R., Norman, G. J., & Meier, D. E. (2018). A study of family caregiver burden and the imperative of practice change to address family caregivers' unmet needs. *Health Affairs Blog*. Retrieved from https://www.healthaffairs.org/do/10.1377/hblog20180105.914873/full/

Thurston, A., Fettig, L., & Arnold, R. (2016). Team communication in the acute care setting. In E. Wittenberg, B. Ferrell, J. Goldsmith, T. Smith, S. L. Ragan, M. Glajchen, & G. Handzo (Eds.), *Textbook of palliative care communication* (pp. 321–329). New York, NY: Oxford University Press.

Trevino, K. M., Prigerson, H. G., Shen, M. J., Tancredi, D. J., Xing, G., Hoerger, M., . . . Duberstein, P. R. (2019). Association between advanced cancer patient–caregiver agreement regarding prognosis and hospice enrollment. *Cancer, 125*(18), 3259–3265. https://doi.org/10.1002/cncr.32188

van Wijngaarden, E., van der Wedden, H., Henning, Z., Komen, R., & The, A. M. (2018). Entangled in uncertainty: The experience of living with dementia from the perspective of family caregivers. *PLoS One, 13*(6), e0198034. https://doi.org/10.1371/journal.pone.0198034

Whitehead, L., Jacob, E., Towell, A., Abu-Qamar, M., & Cole-Heath, A. (2018). The role of the family in supporting the self-management of chronic conditions: A qualitative systematic review. *Journal of Clinical Nursing, 27*(1–2), 22–30. https://doi.org/10.1111/jocn.13775

Wieczorek, C. C., Nowak, P., Frampton, S. B., & Pelikan, J. M. (2018). Strengthening patient and family engagement in healthcare: The New Haven recommendations. *Patient and Education Counseling, 101*(8), 1508–1513. https://doi.org/10.1016/j.pec.2018.04.003

Wittenberg-Lyles, E., Goldsmith, J., & Ragan, S. (2011). The shift to early palliative care: A typology of illness journeys and the role of nursing. *Clinical Journal of Oncology Nursing, 15*(3), 304–310. https://doi.org/10.1188/11.CJON.304-310

World Health Organization. (2018, February 19). *Palliative care: Key facts*. Retrieved from https://www.who.int/news-room/fact-sheets/detail/palliative-care

4

The Family Caregiver Communication Typology

You Can't Unsee Things
February smells like disinfectant, like emptiness and saline. It smells muddled and bitter and barren. February is a sterile hospital room with a once vibrant mother radiated until her marrow dissolves into nothing. A continuous flow of a Saint's platelets and red blood cells to tide her over until the new, unpolluted marrow arrives in an igloo cooler. She takes my latex gloved hand, her tongue swollen and lips cracked and says, "I'm scared." I sit frozen in a moment not knowing how to respond. Disjointed from my body, I'm faintly aware I'm supposed to say something comforting and strong to at least indicate I'm able to console. But time, as though moving through molasses, brings nothing to my bramble-filled thoughts. I squeeze her hand and force a weak smile through stacked up tears, "I know" I say, "Me too."

—Jennifer George Davidson, daughter

Caregiving is not a unified event or task experienced by everyone in the same way. The caregiving experience is as diverse as the care recipient, the caregiver, and the family system to which they all belong. There is constant change, unforeseen activities, progress, and failure along the way that includes a range of events and emotions. The nature and outcome of caregiving and the caregiver's role is shaped by social factors that create circumstances, settings, and pathways of care. A palliative care approach focuses on the social factors that shape caregiver communication patterns and health literacy. Strong, regular, repeated family patterns can create communication burden and influence caregiver health literacy. Chronic illness in the family can force patterns to change or there can be a struggle to maintain existing patterns. When healthcare providers seek to learn what existed before the illness for the patient and family caregiver, they are endowed with the knowledge to provide tailored communication to better meet their health literacy needs. This chapter details how the family system influences a caregiver's communication and caregiving experience, demonstrating the need for an integrated and tailored approach to care for the family caregiver. We introduce four different *family caregiver communication types*, which aid in understanding a caregiver's communication needs and preferences.

CHRONIC ILLNESS AS A STRESSOR TO THE FAMILY SYSTEM

When chronic illness is present for one family member, it has a significant ripple effect throughout the family system. Family rules and patterns, the day-to-day ways of living and functioning as a family, are threatened by the uncertainty of change and must be clarified or altered (Zhang, 2018). The ability of the caregiver to adjust to the stress of the caregiving role produces either a commitment to "standard operating procedure" for family behavior (e.g., we still don't talk about those things no matter the situation or circumstance) or a struggle to reorganize family rules and routines to adjust (Zhang, 2018). In both situations, communication can be uncomfortable for the caregiver as family behaviors are challenged and responses to new communication behaviors are unknown. Positive and negative things occur as family members navigate discussions across "new" family topics and engage in high-stake family decision-making (Rosland et al., 2012).

In many ways, the chronic illness experience brings awareness to the patterns and ways of living for the family; families become more aware of the present ("the way we do things") while keeping an eye on the future ("changes to the way we do things"). Living in the present can require new communication patterns in which talk about illness must occur as part of the adjustment to family functioning (Arestedt et al., 2014). For example, advance care planning discussions are not always topics that families talk about—and then when family members are asked to talk about these topics, most family members are reluctant. Conversations within families about advance care planning are difficult because they create discomfort; caregivers may fear upsetting the patient or feel that they can't broach the subject because the patient isn't feeling well (Schubart et al., 2018). Even when caregivers report that they want to discuss advance care planning, and they believe the patient wants to discuss it with them, they still do not broach the issue (Schubart et al., 2018).

There is an overall tendency for family members to avoid the discomfort of talking about illness, mostly because the uncertainty of illness is perceived to be a threat to the family system (Kuang & Wilson, 2017). Some families may fear that talk about illness and aspects of caregiving may reflect badly on members of the family (Caughlin, 2003), triggering family conflict, or feelings of guilt (Periyakoil et al., 2016). This can result in a hesitation to engage in difficult conversations as well as the tendency to avoid communication. Competing needs or preferences for communication, perceiving insufficient assistance from family members, difficulty agreeing, and different styles of coping and emotional expressiveness all contribute to family communication barriers (Lichtenthal & Kissane, 2008). The following aspects of the family system influence the caregiving experience and can create communication burden encountered by caregivers.

FAMILY EXPECTATIONS FOR CAREGIVING

As a society, families have always been considered the main source for support and assistance when a family member is ill. Among some cultures, family world views influence who in the family is responsible for providing care. For example, the role of caregiver is an expected part of life passed down from generation to generation among Asian American, Hispanic American, and African American caregivers (Pharr et al., 2014). One woman caring for her grandmother with Alzheimer's disease explained:

> I'm Filipino . . . In Tagalog "untagalog no'ob" which means that you owe it to them, like from your inside. Like your soul, you owe it to them. Usually it's the woman's responsibility to take care of the elders in the family. So, filial piety is a thing that's very prominent in Asian culture. The men are also expected to take care of the women, usually women to take care of the elders or like the sick people in your family. But usually it's the women who do it.

Cultural beliefs emphasize family roles for caregiving, and strong cultural feelings for family care directly influence expectations about caregiving (Powers & Whitlatch, 2016).

A caregiver with a sense of duty to care for family members may not find it culturally appropriate to talk about the stress of caregiving or to ask for help. When there is high obligation to help a family member who is ill, there is greater caregiver anxiety and avoidance about the illness (Lee et al., 2017). A deep moral obligation to provide care within the family can motivate caregivers to take on a variety of roles (Reigada et al., 2015), and a strong cultural justification for caregiving may limit requests for assistance from other family members or accepting help from others outside of the family.

FAMILY DECISION-MAKING

The family's ability to make decisions, identify trials and resolve problems is challenged during chronic illness care. When problems related to caregiving cannot be solved (Zhang, 2018), it is often due to long-standing communication barriers present within the family structure and the use of avoidance as a family practice (Wittenberg-Lyles, Demiris, et al., 2012). Communication difficulties among family members occur frequently because of differing communication styles and re-emergence of previous conflicts (Friedermann & Buckwalter, 2014;

Northouse, 2012). Historically hostile relationships can limit family members from engaging in caregiving responsibilities (Wittenberg-Lyles, Demiris, et al., 2012). Some families work to avoid conflict (Anderson & White, 2018). Long-held family communication patterns may remain intact, and a family member who was not communicating with other family members prior to a diagnosis is unlikely to begin communicating with the family after the diagnosis (Bowen et al., 2017).

FAMILY CAREGIVER AND PATIENT RELATIONSHIP

Caregivers often share decision-making with patients or make decisions on the patient's behalf (Given et al., 2012; McCarthy, 2011; Siminoff et al., 2008), placing high importance on the quality of communication between caregiver and care recipient. Conversations between the caregiver and care recipient can vary over time in terms of openness, topics discussed, and specific details shared and is dependent on the dyad's relationship (Goldsmith & Miller, 2014). Patients and caregivers may discuss a range of topics about illness, including pain and bother-some symptoms, medication side effects, trouble paying for care costs, and confusion over healthcare provider instructions (Lee et al., 2017).

When caregivers have a strong relationship with the patient, they are more involved in their care (Lamore et al., 2017), and caregiver–care receiver communication patterns are already in place based on the shared history in the relationship. Among intimate couples, three patterns have been identified (Buck et al., 2018), and each pattern presents unique family system dynamics for the caregiver. First, the active and passive partnership pattern is characterized by a consistent relational pattern wherein one person is more active and the other more passive. If the caregiver is the passive relational partner, then she may feel a need to obtain care recipient permission to seek support and assistance from others for caregiving (Wittenberg-Lyles, Washington et al., 2014). If the caregiver is the active relational partner, then she may feel a need to make decisions on behalf of the patient and lead the decision-making (Laidsaar-Powell et al., 2016). Family caregivers may have different goals than the care recipient and may need help understanding their role as a patient advocate and their identity as a support person in the decision-making process (Lamore et al., 2017).

A second relational pattern emphasizes that everything is achieved together as a couple, with equal footing between care receiver and caregiver. In these dyads, the caregiver serves as a source of emotional support, providing a safe place for sharing the emotional impact of illness (Lamore et al., 2017). In this relational pattern, care recipient and caregiver are more able and willing to discuss topics that extend beyond physical care and treatment. Caregivers work to minimize or manage patient suffering by providing emotional support, keeping the patient's hope up, carrying out the patient's wishes, and communicating empathy and understanding (Reigada et al., 2015). Assistance is needed to help caregivers facilitate the patient's coping as well as their own.

Finally, the last pattern depicts a time when the patient was and could be more active but now relies on the caregiver as a new pattern. Buck et al. (2018) describe how a "patient managed day-to-day pattern" can move into a "caregiver-managed crisis mode" of care. Caregivers become responsible for the patient, participate in decision-making processes that are not about their own health, and must work to be informed (Reigada et al., 2015). This represents a new role within the care recipient–caregiver relationship, as well as the caregiving role in general. Loss of the care recipient as a source of social support can also make it difficult for the caregiver to make decisions (Wittenberg-Lyles, Washington et al., 2014). Family members who serve as surrogates are typically identified because of their special relationship with the patient (Nelson et al., 2017).

FAMILY ROLES

Living with chronic illness is an ongoing process that requires creating alternative ways of living (Arestedt et al., 2014), triggering new family roles within the family system. The person with illness may not be able to continue fulfilling specific family roles, leaving other family members to take on additional responsibilities. Likewise, the demands of caregiving may mean that caregivers will not be able to fulfill roles within routine family life (Zhang, 2018). As a result, family roles and responsibilities can shift and are reallocated among other members. This shift can bring about significant changes in who leads or influences the family.

Changes to family roles sometimes give individual family members more power and other times remove power within the family structure (Mollerberg et al., 2017). For the family member who is ill, power can be gained by becoming the focal point of family decision-making. Family adaptations can include doing more activities at home and adopting a slower pace (Arestedt et al., 2014). Family members may feel compelled to increase time spent with a person with chronic illness. For the care recipient, there can be incredible loss of power as he or she is unable to maintain identity in the family identity (e.g., as breadwinner or child caretaker) and/or fulfill family roles and may feel embarrassed to ask for help with activities of daily living (Gabriel et al., 2014).

Family members may change their way of interacting with one another during illness (Mollerberg et al., 2017). Some family members may avoid the person with chronic illness because they are uncomfortable (Arestedt et al., 2014), leaving care tasks falling to one person. Unequal family engagement in care can create conflict when one person feels like the others are not helping (Anderson & White, 2018). Seeking support from other family members is considered one of the hardest parts of caregiving (Wittenberg-Lyles, Washington et al., 2014). Still, caregiving struggles can be made worse by the family system (Anderson & White, 2018) especially when two caregivers are present and must agree on patient care (Wittenberg-Lyles, Kruse et al., 2014). As a consequence of caregiving, family roles and relationships will be altered, with some getting stronger and others becoming weaker (Arestedt et al., 2014).

FAMILY UNCERTAINTY

When uncertainty about illness is high, there is a tendency to avoid talking about the illness; keeping concerns from each other can become a new family pattern or fortify patterns already in place (Kuang & Wilson, 2017; Mollerberg et al., 2017). For example, family caregivers of lung cancer patients reported that avoiding the topic of cancer was one way of maintaining family standards, recognizing that the family's history of communication influenced how they communicated about cancer (Caughlin et al., 2011). Topic avoidance is often used as a communication strategy aimed at protecting oneself, a relational partner, or a relationship (Ebersole & Hernandez, 2016). Limited communication can occur within families out of fear of the effect that the illness news will have on the patient, fear of inappropriate information given to the patient by the healthcare team, and a family belief that the patient should not be aware of the full extent of her diagnosis/prognosis (Ehsani et al., 2016). Avoiding the topic is a communication strategy that protects the family from the discomfort of talking about death (Basinger et al., 2016). Yet this protective caregiving behavior, when stress is hidden or concealed from the patient, has negative effects on patients (Kayser et al., 2018).

FAMILY COMMUNICATION PATTERNS THEORY

Family communication patterns theory provides a framework for understanding family communication during chronic illness and gives shape to the communication patterns of caregivers. The theory is rooted in family relationship schemas, defined as an individual's cognition of a collectively shared reality, which reveal the interpersonal scripts or family rules for communicating (Fitzpatrick & Ritchie, 1994; McLeod & Chaffee, 1973; Ritchie & Fitzpatrick, 1990). These family rules are governed by two family beliefs regarding conformity and conversation, with each dimension of communication representing a high and low end.

First, *conformity orientation* refers to the degree of family homogeneity wherein the family focuses on uniform beliefs, a priority on family harmony, and obedience to parents/elders (Koerner & Fitzpatrick, 2002). *High conformity orientation* families are characterized by interactions that emphasize and stress harmony, conflict avoidance, and the importance of family communication. These families are considered a traditional family structure due to their focus on cohesion and reliance on hierarchy (Koerner & Fitzpatrick, 2002). Family members prioritize family time over personal time and expect resources to be shared among family members; parents are expected to make decisions for their children (Koerner & Fitzpatrick, 2002). *Low conformity orientation* families stress the importance of independence from family and heterogeneous attitudes and beliefs. Family members view relationships outside the family as equal to family relationships; they value personal space and personal interests (Koerner & Fitzpatrick, 2002).

The second family belief that impacts family communication is *conversation orientation*, the degree to which families create a communication climate. This climate is characterized by free expression and free, spontaneous interaction between family members without limitation of topic or time spent communicating (Fitzpatrick, 2004). Families that have *high conversation orientation* spend a lot of time together, uphold high levels of self-disclosure within the family, and readily engage in family decision-making. Families with high conversation orientation share a joint belief that rewarding family life is a result of frequent and open communication (Koerner & Fitzpatrick, 2002). On the other hand, families that have *low conversation orientation* spend less time together and restrict topics of discussion within the family, such that family decision-making is more likely to occur on an individual or dyadic basis. Typically, these families do not believe that frequent communication is essential to the function of the family (Koerner & Fitzpatrick, 2002).

According to family communication patterns theory, these two beliefs interact with each other to form a family communication pattern. These two dimensions paired in four quadrants reveal four different family types. *Consensual* families are high in both conversation orientation and conformity orientation. Families negotiate the tension between agreeing and preserving hierarchy within the family, yet still are able to freely explore new ideas (Koerner & Fitzpatrick, 2002). With an emphasis on hierarchy, parent–child communication in this family type is characterized by parental decision-making and an emphasis on explaining decisions to the children.

Bert and Mac, a married couple showcased in a PBS documentary *Caring for Your Parents*, are cared for by their four daughters and are an example of a consensual family (Kirk, 2008). Their four daughters reflect on the family process that took place when their parents began to show signs of decline:

> KATHY: We have, as a group, talked several years ago with Mom about when we realized that Dad was losing some ground, what would be next.
>
> JOYCE: I think that was a really important step for all of us to sit and do all of that.
>
> PAT: Clarifying advance directives. Um, you know, things like that.
>
> JOYCE: We needed to know, uh, the insurance policies, the deed to the house, their will. My parents explained if they were ill and in the hospital what kind of life support they would want. We asked, "Oh, would you want a feeding tube?" And they both said no, not a feeding tube to prolong life. So those are important things to know.
>
> ALBERTA: Everybody was feeling okay about it. It took a load off my shoulders, because at that point my husband was not able to help me make good judgments.
>
> JOYCE: It was good that we were all together so that I didn't have to report to you [other sisters] what anybody else said, you didn't have to report to me, so we were all together, we heard the same things at the same

time and then we talked and clarified with each other what's your understanding of that, we're really clear on that, so . . .

PAT: I think it's extremely important to write it down. There's always going
to be some dissension if the family doesn't get it and read it and talk
about it. There will always be dissension.

This reflective account is an exemplar of the communication patterns present in
consensual families. Joyce's comment that it was "important for all of us to sit
and do all of that" highlights the emphasis on family communication as well as
the importance of family conformity. Bert and Mac communicated their wishes
to their children in a formal process, clarifying any questions, and ensuring
that all children were present and equally represented in the decision-making
process.

Pluralistic families are high in conversation orientation and low in conformity
orientation. These families have open discussions that involve all family members,
and parents do not necessarily make all decisions for the children. Pluralistic
families value participatory decision-making that includes their children's
opinions, valuing the merit of an argument rather than the family member who
presents the argument (Koerner & Fitzpatrick, 2002). The mother of a 28-year-old
terminally ill daughter explained how her family decided on an inpatient hospice
facility instead of home care:

So anyway we are at that point [deciding on placement]. I'll need to move
her on Friday. I had really thought that I would take her home, but my older
daughter asked me not to do it. She said I could never come over and sleep
the night or be in this room knowing [name] died in this room. And I have
to respect her; she's losing her best friend [crying].

For this family, it was important for everyone's input to be considered and for
their opinion to influence family decision-making. This family clearly had a discussion about this important decision, and the daughter's feelings about the situation were valued even more than the mother's own feelings.

On the other hand, *protective* families are low on conversation orientation and
high on conformity orientation. These families rely heavily on obedience to parental authority and engage in very little communication. Parents make decisions
and do not need to explain their reasoning or rationale to their children (Koerner
& Fitzpatrick, 2002). Bonnie, who was handling her mother's care, recalls the day
she and her mother learned that her mother had cancer:

INTERVIEWER: So did he [doctor], did he communicate in that meeting that
she would not ever live without the cancer? I mean was that clear? That
wasn't clear?

BONNIE: No, it was like the next step, chemo or radiation or whatever.

INTERVIEWER: So what do you think she [mother] thought?

BONNIE: I don't know, she didn't say. You know, we didn't talk about it. We really didn't discuss it. The thing we discussed was the next appointment and the next doctor. And who was going to you know, be there . . .

Bonnie's experience highlights the conforming nature of the protective family communication pattern. Rather than discussing the prognosis, Bonnie followed her mother's direction and began making arrangements for the next doctor visit. She did not even consider talking more about the topic with her mother.

Finally, *laissez-faire* families are low in both conversation orientation and conformity orientation. This family type is characterized by very little interaction between family members and emotional detachment. Upon arrival to a hospice inpatient facility, a woman, dying from esophageal cancer (Pt), was asked about her family by the nurse (RN):

RN: How is your family doing with all of this?
PT: None of them are talking to me.
RN: They might be afraid—you might need to bring it up.
PT: Yes they are.
RN: [long pause] You might need to bring it up.
PT: I have a niece and nephew. I haven't seen them in two years and they live right here in town. They said they were coming yesterday and they didn't. But maybe I was sleeping. I feel like they are using it as an excuse, but I don't care if they have an excuse now. I was not the most popular person in my family. I'm the oldest and I've always had to do the most and sometimes it put me in an unpopular position. I was the tattle-tale. Mommy and Daddy expected me to report everything.

For many laissez-faire family types, a chronic illness diagnosis for a family member prompts a reason for communication when no reason for communication existed before. Interestingly, this woman provides a rationale for the limited communication that has taken place, blaming her own position and role within her family.

When a family member is diagnosed with a chronic illness, family communication patterns are highlighted by the illness crisis. The four family types (consensual, pluralistic, protective, laissez-faire) inform the patterns. We extended these ideas offered in the theory to illustrate how caregivers vary in the ways that they talk about illness with the patient, family, and healthcare providers. Next, we describe the development of the Family Caregiver Communication Typology.

DEVELOPMENT OF THE FAMILY CAREGIVER COMMUNICATION TYPOLOGY

Variance in interaction patterns between family members exists and greatly impacts the caregiver (Nissen et al., 2016; Schuler et al., 2014). As previously reviewed, family expectations for caregiving, family decision-making, family caregiver and patient relationship, family roles, and family uncertainty all contribute to the caregiving experience and the communication burden of the caregiver. Initially we conducted a theoretical exploration of the stress and coping of caregivers. We analyzed 81 hospice caregivers and their discussion about caregiving problems and found that family communication is a secondary stressor for caregivers (Wittenberg-Lyles, Demiris, et al., 2012). Using the theory as a framework, we explored audio-recorded discussions of caregiving problems during a six-week period of time with 126 hospice caregivers. Our analysis of these discussions revealed four specific communication patterns among caregivers: Manager, Carrier, Partner, and Lone (Wittenberg-Lyles, Goldsmith, Demiris, et al., 2012).

Figure 4.1 depicts how each caregiver type is embedded/grounded in one of the four family communication patterns. While high and low patterns reflect communication within family systems, the context of communication (in this volume, the context is caregiving in chronic illness) is further discerned through warm and cold levels of communication (Hesse et al., 2017). COLD conformity occurs when one member uses family obligation to exert control and influence over another, preventing or hindering open conversations and debate and isolating family members from outside influences (Hesse et al., 2017). Families with HIGH/COLD conformity may require a family member to serve as caregiver, place high expectations on caregiving responsibilities, restrict a family members' role solely to caregiving responsibilities, limit their ability to engage in outside time, and restrict conversation about other values. LOW/COLD conformity families experience inconsistent rules about family roles when someone is ill, when there is an inequity of resources, and when there is no featured core value for caring

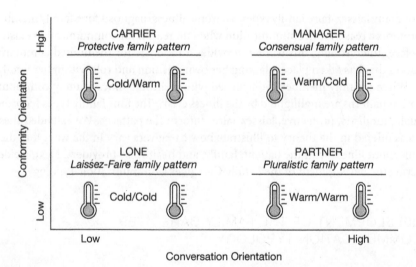

Figure 4.1. Four family caregiver communication types based on the family communication patterns theory constructs of conversation and conformity. © Comfort Communication Project.

for family members. The absence of fixed structures to share in family illness experiences makes the cultivation of closeness in this family almost nonexistent.

WARM conformity, on the other hand, involves consistency in upholding rules, shared beliefs that include equity, designated family times, and a value of family closeness (Hesse et al., 2017). During illness, family obligation draws other members to the tasks and responsibilities of performing family. Caregivers from families with HIGH/WARM conformity have rules about spending time with the ill family member and clear expectations for coming together when a family member has a health crisis; the caregiver's responsibility includes monitoring family involvement to remain connected and communicating family values centered on closeness (Hesse et al., 2017). In a LOW/WARM conformity pattern there are no rules for spending time with the ill family member, only that support is expected. The modality of the support is not prescriptive nor are there set expectations for the timing of that support.

There are also warm and cold levels of conversation patterns. COLD conversation occurs when there is infrequent interaction and limited conversation about a topic that serves to create distance among family members. Caregivers from HIGH/COLD conversation families are supported by family members who share an expectation to agree during illness conversations and conceal differences of opinion. There are clear rules for what can be discussed about illness, to what depth, and when these discussions can occur. In LOW/COLD conversation, there are no expectations for conversation between family members during illness or otherwise and thus no expectations for agreement between caregiver and care recipient.

WARM conversation occurs when communication among family members is a significant and dedicated activity, producing regular contact that includes both a broad range of topics and depth of discussion among multiple family members. Caregivers from HIGH/WARM conversation families have few restrictions about what can be discussed about the illness, when it can happen, and the depth of these discussions. There are no rules for conversation about illness between family members and topics can include emotion, conflict, stress, etc. In LOW/WARM conversation, there are unclear rules for communication about illness, and topic range and depth can vary. Family members, including the caregiver, are inhibited in their engagement with each other and permissible topics and timing are allowed only when they function to preserve family.

Building the Typology

With four caregiver communication types outlined (Manager, Carrier, Partner, Lone), we next applied the four types to video-recorded sessions between family caregivers and interdisciplinary hospice providers (Wittenberg-Lyles, Goldsmith, Oliver, et al., 2012). Each caregiver type demonstrated essential communication traits with a range of providers. Then, we reviewed a clinical case study of a husband and wife who were both afflicted with stage IV cancer; both were performing caregiving duties, and both were facing concentric circles of burden (Goldsmith et al., 2011). Within the same family system, family members can have different caregiver communication types. Next, national audiences of clinicians ($n = 466$) were exposed to the typology, confirming face validity from providers (Wittenberg, Ferrell, Goldsmith, Ragan et al., 2017).

We explored the patient–caregiver dyad to ensure that caregiver communication type was validated both as self-report by caregivers and as perceived by patients. We interviewed 24 dyads (cancer patient and caregiver) separately and concurrently. When asked to identify the caregiver's communication type, cancer patients were likely to identify the same type self-identified by the caregiver (Goldsmith et al., 2016).

To help providers identify caregiver communication types, we developed a 14-item tool based on feedback from an expert review group (experts in the theory, caregiving, communication). We then used this tool to explore the validity of the typology and the impact of communication type and clinical caregiver outcomes. In a pilot sample of 21 caregivers who completed the tool and clinical caregiver outcomes, along with field notes on the family system by an intervention nurse, we reduced the tool to 10 items and found it was 85% accurate (Wittenberg, Kravits, et al., 2017).

Known as the Family Caregiver Communication Tool, this tool measures the frequency, range, and conformity of communication within the patient's family to determine a specific caregiver communication type (Wittenberg, Ferrell, Goldsmith, & Ruel, 2017). The tool and scoring instructions can be found in Box 4.1. Next, we briefly describe each caregiver communication type.

FAMILY CAREGIVER COMMUNICATION TYPOLOGY

Family members share a unique relational history; thus, not all family members are the same family caregiver type (Caughlin et al., 2011; Wittenberg et al., 2017). The emergent caregiver type is dependent upon the relationship between the person with illness and the family caregiver based on communication patterns established over time within the family system. For example, a woman providing care to her mother would likely exhibit a different communication type if providing care to her sister. Each caregiver type depicts unique communication characteristics specific to her or his family communication pattern and has both strengths and weaknesses. We return to our four caregivers (introduced in Chapters 1 and 2 of this volume) and the person they care for (introduced in Chapter 3 of this volume) by describing the dynamics of their family context and revealing their family caregiver communication type. We note here that any caregiver type can experience any of the illness journeys described in Chapter 3 (isolated, rescued, or comforted) and that the four disease factors (onset of disease, course of disease, outcome of disease, and degree of patient incapacitation) influence a caregiver's journey. These dimensions of caregiver are further explored in the following chapters.

Box 4.1

FAMILY CAREGIVER COMMUNICATION TOOL©

Directions: Family can be your partner and/or children. Family can also be the family you were born into, like your parents/guardians and brothers and sisters. Family can also be a group of people you call family, but may not be related to by blood or the law. As primary caregiver for your loved one, think about the family that is connected to you and your loved one (patient). How many people do you consider to be in your family? ____

1. I talk with my family, which can include online and text messages, about my loved one's illness.

   Frequently (4)   Occasionally (3)   Rarely (2)   Very rarely (1)   Never (0)

2. After a medical appointment, I contact family members to share details of the visit.

   Frequently (4)   Occasionally (3)   Rarely (2)   Very rarely (1)   Never (0)

3. Family members ask me about my loved one's illness.

   Frequently (4)   Occasionally (3)   Rarely (2)   Very rarely (1)   Never (0)

4. My family talks about death and dying with our ill loved one.

   Frequently (4)   Occasionally (3)   Rarely (2)   Very rarely (1)   Never (0)

5. My family talks about what might happen if treatment doesn't work.

   Frequently (4)   Occasionally (3)   Rarely (2)   Very rarely (1)   Never (0)

6. My family lets me know that they expect me to take care of my loved one and that I am to do most of the caregiving.

   Frequently (4)   Occasionally (3)   Rarely (2)   Very rarely (1)   Never (0)

7. When I am stressed from caregiving, I prefer to hide this from family members.

   Frequently (4)   Occasionally (3)   Rarely (2)   Very rarely (1)   Never (0)

8. My family hides their opinion about the quality of my caregiving.

   Frequently (4)   Occasionally (3)   Rarely (2)   Very rarely (1)   Never (0)

9. My family tries to act as though my loved one is not ill.

   Frequently (4)   Occasionally (3)   Rarely (2)   Very rarely (1)   Never (0)

10. My ill loved one lets me know that he/she expects me to provide care and do most of the caregiving.

    Frequently (4)   Occasionally (3)   Rarely (2)   Very rarely (1)   Never (0)

Instructions for Scoring the Family Caregiver Communication Tool

The tool is a valid and reliable instrument for obtaining information about the frequency, range, and congruence of communication within the patient's family. It is composed of two subscales: conversation and conformity. The tool is a 10-item instrument completed by the primary family caregiver about her/his communication with family about the patient's illness and values and beliefs about caregiving. The purpose of the tool is to derive a specific caregiver type. Below are instructions for scoring the tool.

Scoring instructions

A family caregiver type is computed as follows:

1. Add items 1–5 to calculate the score for conversation.
2. Add items 6–10 to calculate the score for conformity.

The maximum range of scores for each subscale of the tool is from 0 to 20, with higher scores indicating a stronger communication pattern.

Interpreting the Score

To determine a caregiver type, use the median score as the cut-off point between the two subscales (0–11 low; 12–20 is high) and interpret the score as follows:

Conversation low, Conformity low—Lone Caregiver
Conversation low, Conformity high—Carrier Caregiver
Conversation high, Conformity low—Partner Caregiver
Conversation high, Conformity high—Manager Caregiver

©Comfort Communication Project, 2020.

Manager Caregiver

In some families there is a natural leader who says "yes" to caregiving. This caregiver manages every aspect of the illness and leads the family in decisions about care. This family role includes speaking up at medical appointments and talking with family about the illness. The patient defers ideas and care decisions to this caregiver, while the family engages in conversation about life around the illness and focuses on the positive. As the family spokesperson, the Manager caregiver values information about the illness and related medical information.

For the Manager caregiver, an active-confrontational communication pattern with physicians is prominent (Peters et al., 2019). There is reliance on "us versus them" in terms of sharing family preferences with providers and an emphasis on things that *must* and *should* be done. Manager caregivers are able to request help from medical staff if needed, actively voicing concerns if they have them, and comfortably and boldly requesting additional information.

The Manager is eager to act, to improve the care situation, and to intervene. The desires of the patient and other family are not directly part of the decision-making process for this caregiver. A focus on the physical care of the patient is also common for the Manager, but this caregiver is also able to see the psychosocial needs of this patient. This caregiver is steeped in the research and medical language of the healthcare world, but her conceptual understanding of those things does not keep pace with the way she presents herself to healthcare providers. For example, she may use the same medical language providers use but she is likely to lack a careful understanding of what those terms mean in the context of her family member's illness.

Maggie Burkhart is a Manager caregiver. Maggie has two sisters and one brother. One sister (Jenny) lives in the same town, one (Judith) lives about three hours away by car, and her brother (Billy) lives several states away. Eight years ago, their dad was diagnosed with an advanced cancer diagnosis and died within 7 months. Their mother, Earlene, remained in the family home on her own, and none of the children lived close to her. Jenny was nearest and had a 45-minute drive to reach Earlene's house. Over a period of about five years, the three daughters pieced together that Earlene was, in fact, living with and compensating mightily for dementia. Jenny became the durable medical power of attorney and found a nursing home for Earlene somewhat closer to Jenny's house. Jenny's focus for Earlene's care emphasized pharmaceutical management.

Once Maggie and Judith realized Earlene was refusing to bathe, was falling regularly, and was in a facility that was unclean and smelled strongly of urine, they wanted to move their mom. It was at this point that Maggie took over the care for their mother. Maggie sees her mom each day and monitors her care and communication with providers very closely. Maggie left her job as a top-level administrator at a nearby educational system to oversee her mom's care.

Jenny has not spoken with her siblings and has not seen her mother in six months, since she moved into a new facility in the town where Maggie and Judith live. Jenny remains the durable medical power of attorney, although the care facility where Earlene stays works with Maggie to make every decision. The oldest child, Billy, has yet to visit his mom in the new nursing facility. With the longevity of caregiving due to dementia and family discord over their mother's care, Maggie and her family will likely experience a rescued journey as Earlene's disease progresses and hospice ultimately becomes involved at the nursing home.

CARRIER CAREGIVER

Sometimes families do not talk directly about the illness and work to avoid conflict. Although family members may be physically present, the Carrier caregiver focuses on protecting others from the burden of caregiving. The patient makes decisions, and this caregiver makes sure that these decisions are put into action. Other family members are in the network of interaction, yet the Carrier caregiver has a hard time accepting or asking for help from other network members and feels a deep sense of family obligation to serve as caregiver.

The Carrier caregiver exhibits a passive-cooperative communication pattern with physicians (Peters et al., 2019). This caregiver has a strong need to demonstrate agreement, trusting healthcare providers and avoiding explicit discussions about the nature of the illness. Typically, Carrier caregivers state that they are uncertain about medical terms and prefer to leave decision-making to providers. The Carrier will not find support and comfort within the family structure. Carrier caregivers are surrounded by other family who could ameliorate the load, but the family dynamics do not allow for roles to shift. The Carrier finds support and solace in healthcare providers and will rely on them for support and decision-making help. Recommendations for patient care are guided heavily by providers, determined by the patient, and executed by the caregiver.

Sharon Jenks is a Carrier caregiver. Sharon and Kelley are in a life partnership. Also part of this family is Joan, Kelley's 89-year old mom. They all reside in a large western city in the United States. Following her mesothelioma cancer diagnosis, Kelley ultimately pursued six lines of chemotherapeutic treatments. She stopped working one year into her diagnosed illness and had little strength to participate in activities she enjoyed. She spent most of her time at home recovering from treatment. Kelley and Sharon saw their pursuit of curative therapies as the most productive and promising approach to combat the illness.

Sharon finds herself in a family system that has a lot of people in it with a lot of expectations, and she works to fulfill every need and request of Kelley, the care recipient. Kelley calls the shots and Sharon works tirelessly to be her hands and feet and even to take on the responsibilities of Kelley—essentially burning all of her own energy on behalf of the patient and the rest of the family.

Exactly two years from her diagnosis, Kelley died. It was an isolated journey as there was no palliative or hospice care included in her medical treatment. The authors have very little detail about her final days and the experience of the family. Joan (mother) and Sharon (partner) remain embroiled in a financial conflict that centers on Kelley's care decisions and life insurance. The two are currently unwilling to communicate about Kelley's final experience due to this conflict.

PARTNER CAREGIVER

For the Partner, caregiving often includes more than one caregiver. For some, caregiving may derive from many players in the family contributing, including the patient. Everyone actively contributes what they can to share caregiving labors. Family members talk openly about caregiving and share different ideas. Disagreements happen, conflict can rage, and then solutions are determined within the family. The patient and the family are concerned about the well-being of the Partner caregiver and integrate their needs into care management.

The Partner caregiver enjoys an active-cooperative communication pattern with physicians (Peters et al., 2019). Frequently using medical terminology that matches healthcare providers, the Partner caregiver readily expresses emotional experiences and has a positive attitude toward medical staff. Partner caregivers feel secure and request some information from providers but mainly rely on external sources of information from within their social network.

Estella Rodriguez is a Partner caregiver. Her father, Marco, was diagnosed with advanced stage multiple myeloma. She and her siblings identified roles in the caregiving process and shifted into action to assist their parents. The roles were adjusted multiple times as they became more and more familiar with their parents' needs. Estella became researcher and planner. Her sister became the financial consultant, and her two brothers were hands-on caregivers and comforters to their parents. At this late stage of illness, Marco's vertebrae and ribs were breaking even during minimal movement. His pain level soared, and by the fall, he was incapacitated and bed-ridden. By winter, Marco had deteriorated substantially, and his pain was protracted and unceasing. A referral to a regional healthcare center for a stem cell transplant put this family on an accidental course to acquiring palliative care, affording the family a comforted journey.

Following the family's consultation with a palliative care team, the reason for Marco's initial referral, the stem-cell transplant was put on hold until his quality of life could be improved. By spring, due to pain relief, nutrition care, therapies, and communication with a medical care team, Marco moved from a wheelchair, to a walker, to a cane in his ambulation, and experienced complete pain relief. A year from the start of his illness journey, Marco and his wife had become fully independent in their own home once again. No household or medical caretakers are currently needed. Their children remain involved and realistic about their Dad's prognosis and are wary of Marco's choice to withdraw from palliative care and return to his previous oncologist in his hometown.

The Partner caregiver featured in this family, Estella, is situated in a family that navigates differences and changes with flexibility. As roles shift, the members of the family care team shift, providing shared relief for the primary caregiver. The patient's wishes and needs weigh heavily in the care decisions and practices undertaken by this caregiver. The family is a safe place for support, troubles telling, and sharing about caregiving stressors. This kind of caregiver regularly encounters differences of opinion and conflict, but the communication climate of this family allows for navigation of difficulties. The effect of having many engaged and weight-bearing family members involved in care presents a "too many cooks in the kitchen" dynamic. Not everyone will know what is going on, where the care is taking place, and who the providers are. No one party has the whole story or care plan in this family.

LONE CAREGIVER

Family size does not matter when it comes to caregiving. Nestled in a family of five, a caregiver may be on his own in providing care and making decisions. The patient relies on a Lone caregiver for information, care, and emotional support—in short, everything. As a result, the caregiver has many concerns because the patient has many needs. It is not uncommon for the caregiver to feel frustration or even anger, resentment, and abandonment because the family is not helping more. The Lone caregiver feels as if little help is available, with little energy to do anything other than caregiving.

The Lone caregiver explicitly notes high uncertainty and seeks support and guidance from ongoing relationships with providers. While this caregiver expresses strong preference for agreement, the Lone caregiver also questions professional decisions or errors that occur due to a lack of thoroughness in the medical system. Decision-making is primarily undertaken between the caregiver and staff, and the patient and caregiver are often tightly partnered in the management and navigation of care. Lone caregivers continually request more information but ultimately rely on doctors as the only source of acceptable information.

Viv Gray is a Lone caregiver. She met Jake many years ago, before his time in the Gulf War, and when he was actively drinking. They became partners as he became sober, reaching out to each other via social media, and they have now been together many years. Jake's illnesses have left both Jake and Viv to depend only on each other. Jake was one of the youngest people in the military ever diagnosed with gout. This was followed by injuries in training. But his combat experience in the Middle East was the creator of his posttraumatic stress disorder. Fifteen years of addictions were an effective cover for his chronic illnesses. Once those were removed, his healthcare started in earnest, as did his decline in health. Now on disability at the age of 48, Jake is chasing care and relief for several chronic conditions, the most recent of which is type 2 diabetes.

Viv works very hard to find care providers, navigate the Veterans Affairs system, and pursue avenues within the system to help Jake find relief and quality care. She is most often very dissatisfied with the providers they see and spends copious amounts of time looking for treatments and pathways online. She has no social life. Jake occupies the time that would otherwise be given to rest, creative projects, travel, and social life. She has minimal support coming mostly from two friends at work who know little about the burden of caring for Jake. Lone caregivers are very much alone. Their interaction and decision-making about Jake's health takes place in and around the healthcare system; they have little social or familial support. Families surrounding the patient are distant and uninvolved, even if they live across the street. These caregivers know a lot about places of care and providers and are heavily focused on the biomedical fires in their midst. The psychosocial elements of chronic illness are less central to their labors of finding care.

WHY FAMILY CAREGIVING TYPES MATTER

Up until this point, we have established the imperative to care for the family caregiver in chronic illness, the need to understand the family system to overcome health literacy barriers, and how the involvement of palliative care or a palliative care approach to communication about chronic illness can promote caregiver understanding of disease and its trajectory. Improving caregiver communication and health literacy is essential in supporting the caregiver and has the potential to influence both patient and caregiver outcomes.

A caregiver's information and health literacy needs have a direct impact on patient care. Caregivers do not currently receive enough information and education to support their caregiving role (Grant et al., 2013; Meeker et al., 2011), and unmet information needs about illness, treatment, and care-related information are associated with patient physical symptoms, anxiety, and quality of life (Wang et al., 2018). Adverse effects of caregiver health literacy barriers on patient outcomes include misunderstanding prescription medication directions, inadequate knowledge of cancer and treatment effects (US Department of Health and Human Services, 2018), inability to assist with safe and effective home medication use (Roter et al., 2018), and risk of hospital readmission for the patient (Rodakowski et al., 2017). Moreover, poor caregiver mental and physical health impacts the ability to communicate productively with clinical staff (Litzelman et al., 2016). Ineffective communication between clinicians and caregivers impedes caregiver learning (Lau et al., 2010) and can result in poor adherence that leaves patient pain undertreated (Mayahara, 2011; Miaskowski et al., 2001).

Family communication about chronic illness (or lack of communication about chronic illness) influences the caregiver's ability to communicate with the care recipient and providers, which impacts patient care (Rosland et al., 2012). Within the family, family self-reliance and cohesion are associated with better patient outcomes (Ewing et al., 2016). When a family caregiver can provide informational, emotional, and instrumental support tailored to the person with chronic illness, patient outcomes such as readmission rates, emergency department presentations, and anxiety levels improve (Deek et al., 2016). Likewise, patients who do not feel a sense of support from within their family experience more stress and anxiety, worry more, have lower self-efficacy, and have a lower sense of assurance about palliative care (Milberg et al., 2014).

When caregiver health literacy needs are met and palliative care support is provided that helps caregivers to communicate more openly about chronic illness, caregiver and patient outcomes improve. The caregiver's ability to find information and ask for help is a key factor in obtaining supportive resources for caregiving tasks (Ferrell & Wittenberg, 2017; Northouse et al., 2010), and having additional resources lowers caregiver stress (Empeno et al., 2011). Improving the caregiver's ability to talk about cancer mediates coping and positively impacts the stress process (Fletcher et al., 2012). The ability and willingness to share information about cancer improves patient quality of life (Lai et al., 2017) and enhances relational quality between patient and caregiver, which lowers caregiver depressive symptoms (Hou et al., 2018).

Early evidence demonstrates that caregiver effectiveness and well-being can be improved by palliative care support. Educational sessions that include communication reduce caregiver burden (Cianfrocca et al., 2018), improve caregiver quality of life and relational intimacy (Borneman et al., 2015), and make caregivers more conscious of their role and the importance of their actions as they relate to caregiver quality of life and patient outcomes (Cianfrocca et al., 2018). To truly enact a tailored a patient-centered approach to care, the family caregiver must be included.

Thus, the provider's ability to discern a family caregiver communication type has great significance. Family caregiver communication types influence caregiver stress and burden during caregiving, and there is variance in caregiver outcomes among the four types (Wittenberg, Kravits, et al., 2017). Caregiver types also exhibit specific communication behaviors with healthcare providers (Wittenberg-Lyles, Goldsmith, Oliver, et al., 2012) and indicate that the level of caregiver participation in shared decision-making is influenced by provider communication. If the family caregiver is able to access, understand, and use information about the illness in communicating about it with the patient, family, and healthcare providers, she is more likely to be successful in caring for the patient and herself.

The typology provides an in-depth understanding of the variance found in caregiving outcomes. A preponderance of research on family caregiving has concluded that caregivers share a reciprocal experience with the patient and simultaneously experience poor outcomes, lack self-care, and have high information needs. Yet there is little understanding for *why* and *how* this occurs despite healthcare interventions that address and include the family caregiver. *A palliative care approach addresses communication and health literacy burdens, which prohibit caregivers from successfully navigating the healthcare system and assists the care recipient with making informed, shared decisions about chronic illness.* The typology provides a theoretical explanation in the chronic illness literature supported by an evidence that reveals specific and unique reasons for caregiver outcomes. For example, communication burden experienced as a result of LOW/COLD conformity informs providers that the caregiver has only one person with whom to confide caregiver stress, and that is the care recipient. In this scenario, dyadic intervention may be appropriate, whereas a caregiver experiencing burden as a result of HIGH/WARM conformity would benefit most from a family meeting to discuss caregiver stress rather than a dyadic intervention. By learning about caregiver types, providers can best determine appropriate interventions that address communication burden, which can mediate care outcomes.

Second, the inclusion of a palliative care approach by providers illuminates the variance in illness journeys for caregivers, which is also tied to care outcomes. Navigation of the healthcare system and utilization of available support services within the healthcare organization, community, and family are dependent upon the caregiver's communication and health literacy skills. When healthcare providers begin to work with a family caregiver, they need to be knowledgeable about the family system which they are entering. There are differences in the way that caregivers present themselves to others, sometimes as knowledgeable and well-supported. Understanding caregiver communication burden will reveal more accurate health literacy needs of the family caregiver, allowing providers to practice adaptable and flexible communication when caring for the family caregiver.

CONCLUSION

Implementing communication and health literacy strategies for all patients and family caregivers is essential for providing quality palliative care. However, healthcare providers that learn about established family dynamics and communication patterns that have existed long before a patient's chronic illness will be better situated to provide nuanced, caregiver communication and health literacy interventions that align with the specific orientation of a caregiver. Communication is a core construct in the function of family (Beavers & Hampson, 2000; Fitzpatrick, 2004; Olson & Gorall, 2003; Skinner et al., 2000). Sensitive, effective communication is number one among the five major themes central to patients and their family caregiver (Tallman et al., 2012). Chronic illness creates an opportunity for family members to receive support from each other and to talk about things that previously were never talked about (Benzein et al., 2015). As the caregiver typology has grown throughout the last decade, this volume provides a place to discuss our research about the Manager, Partner, Carrier, and Lone caregivers in depth and in context of chronic illness. The exercise of studying each of the types across time and in differing diagnoses has given all four of the types more dimension. As we have peeled back the layers of understanding and knowledge, the elements of conformity and conversation are increasingly more important in helping us describe how communication burden differs between the types and informs tailored communication approaches for providers.

REFERENCES

Anderson, E. W., & White, K. M. (2018). "This is what family does": The family experience of caring for serious illness. *American Journal of Hospice & Palliative Care, 35*(2), 348–354. https://doi.org/10.1177/1049909117709251

Arestedt, L., Persson, C., & Benzein, E. (2014). Living as a family in the midst of chronic illness. *Scandinavian Journal of Caring Science, 28*(1), 29–37. https://doi.org/10.1111/scs.12023

Basinger, E. D., Wehrman, E. C., & McAninch, K. G. (2016). Grief communication and privacy rules: Examining the communication of individuals bereaved by the death of a family member. *Journal of Family Communication, 16*(4), 285–302.

Beavers, H., & Hampson, R. (2000). The Beavers system model of family functioning. *Journal of Family Theory, 22*, 128–143.

Benzein, E., Olin, C., & Persson, C. (2015). "You put it all together": Families' evaluation of participating in family health conversations. *Scandinavian Journal of Caring Science, 29*(1), 136–144. https://doi.org/10.1111/scs.12141

Borneman, T., Sun, V., Williams, A. C., Fujinami, R., Del Ferraro, C., Burhenn, P. S., . . . Buga, S. (2015). Support for patients and family caregivers in lung cancer: Educational components of an interdisciplinary palliative care intervention. *Journal of Hospice & Palliative Nursing, 17*(4), 309–318. https://doi.org/10.1097/NJH.0000000000000165

Bowen, D. J., Hay, J. L., Harris-Wai, J. N., Meischke, H., & Burke, W. (2017). All in the family? Communication of cancer survivors with their families. *Familial Cancer, 16*(4), 597–603. https://doi.org/10.1007/s10689-017-9987-8

Buck, H. G., Hupcey, J., & Watach, A. (2018). Pattern versus change: Community-based dyadic heart failure self-care. *Clinical Nursing Research, 27*(2), 148–161. https://doi.org/10.1177/1054773816688817

Caughlin, J. P. (2003). Family communication standards what counts as excellent family communication and how are such standards associated with family satisfaction? *Human Communication Research, 29*(1), 5–40.

Caughlin, J. P., Mikucki-Enyart, S., Middelton, A., Stone, A., & Brown, L. (2011). Being open without talking about it: A rhetorical/normative approach to understanding topic avoidance in families after a lung cancer diagnosis. *Communication Monographs, 78*(4), 409–436. https://doi.org/10.1080/03637751.2011.618141

Cianfrocca, C., Caponnetto, V., Donati, D., Lancia, L., Tartaglini, D., & Di Stasio, E. (2018). The effects of a multidisciplinary education course on the burden, health literacy and needs of family caregivers. *Applied Nursing Research, 44*, 100–106. https://doi.org/10.1016/j.apnr.2018.10.004

Deek, H., Hamilton, S., Brown, N., Inglis, S. C., Digiacomo, M., Newton, P. J., . . . Davidson, P. M. (2016). Family-centered approaches to healthcare interventions in chronic diseases in adults: A quantitative systematic review. *Journal of Advanced Nursing, 72*(5), 968–979. https://doi.org/10.1111/jan.12885

Ebersole, D. S., & Hernandez, R. A. (2016). "Taking good care of our health": Parent-adolescent perceptions of boundary management about health information. *Communication Quarterly, 64*(5), 573–595.

Ehsani, M., Taleghani, F., Hematti, S., & Abazari, P. (2016). Perceptions of patients, families, physicians and nurses regarding challenges in cancer disclosure: A descriptive qualitative study. *European Journal of Oncology Nursing, 25*, 55–61. https://doi.org/10.1016/j.ejon.2016.09.003

Empeno, J., Raming, N. T., Irwin, S. A., Nelesen, R. A., & Lloyd, L. S. (2011). The hospice caregiver support project: Providing support to reduce caregiver stress. *Journal of Palliative Medicine, 14*(5), 593–597. https://doi.org/10.1089/jpm.2010.0520

Ewing, G., Ngwenya, N., Benson, J., Gilligan, D., Bailey, S., Seymour, J., & Farquhar, M. (2016). Sharing news of a lung cancer diagnosis with adult family members and friends: A qualitative study to inform a supportive intervention. *Patient Education & Counseling, 99*(3), 378–385. https://doi.org/10.1016/j.pec.2015.09.013

Ferrell, B., & Wittenberg, E. (2017). A review of family caregiving intervention trials in oncology. *Cancer, 67*(4), 318–325. https://doi.org/10.3322/caac.21396

Fitzpatrick, M. A. (2004). Family communication patterns theory: Observations on its development and application. *Journal of Family Communication, 4*(3–4), 167–179.

Fitzpatrick, M. A., & Ritchie, L. (1994). Communication schemata within the family: Multiple perspectives on family interaction. *Human Communication Research, 20*, 275–301.

Fletcher, B. S., Miaskowski, C., Given, B., & Schumacher, K. (2012). The cancer family caregiving experience: An updated and expanded conceptual model. *European Journal of Oncology Nursing, 16*(4), 387–398. https://doi.org/10.1016/j.ejon.2011.09.001

Friedermann, M.-L., & Buckwalter, K. (2014). Family caregiver role and burden related to gender and family relationships. *Journal of Family Nursing, 20*(3), 313–336. https://doi.org/10.1177/1074840714532715

Gabriel, R., Figueiredo, D., Jacome, C., Cruz, J., & Marques, A. (2014). Day-to-day living with severe chronic obstructive pulmonary disease: Towards a family-based approach to the illness impacts. *Psychology & Health, 29*(8), 967–983. https://doi.org/10.1080/08870446.2014.902458

Given, B., Given, C., & Sherwood, P. (2012). Family and caregiver needs over the course of the cancer trajectory. *Journal of Supportive Oncology, 10,* 57–64.

Goldsmith, D., & Miller, G. (2014). Conceptualizing how couples talk about cancer. *Health Communication, 29,* 51–63. https://doi.org/10.1080/10410236.2012.717215

Goldsmith, J., Wittenberg, E., Platt, C. S., Iannarino, N. T., & Reno, J. (2016). Family caregiver communication in oncology: Advancing a typology. *Psycho-Oncology, 25*(4), 463–470. https://doi.org/10.1002/pon.3862

Goldsmith, J., Wittenberg-Lyles, E., & Burchett, M. (2011). When patient becomes caregiver: One couple, two cases of advanced cancer. In B. Maria (Ed.), *Contemporary case studies in health communication: Theoretical and applied approaches* (2nd ed., pp. 205–216). Dubuque, IA: Kendall Hunt.

Grant, M., Sun, V., Fujinami, R., Sidhu, R., Otis-Green, S., Juarez, G., . . . Ferrell, B. (2013). Family caregiver burden, skills preparedness, and quality of life in non-small cell lung cancer. *Oncology Nursing Forum, 40*(4), 337–346. https://doi.org/10.1188/13.ONF.337-346

Hesse, C., Rauscher, E. A., Budesky Goodman, R., & Couvrette, M. A. (2017). Reconceptualizing the role of conformity behaviors in family communication patterns theory. *Journal of Family Communication, 17*(4), 319–337.

Hou, W. K., Lau, K. M., Shum, T. C. Y., Cheng, A. C. K., & Lee, T. M. C. (2018). Do concordances of social support and relationship quality predict psychological distress and well-being of cancer patients and caregivers? *European Journal of Cancer Care (Engl), 27*(4), e12857. https://doi.org/10.1111/ecc.12857

Kayser, K., Acquati, C., Reese, J. B., Mark, K., Wittmann, D., & Karam, E. (2018). A systematic review of dyadic studies examining relationship quality in couples facing colorectal cancer together. *Psycho-Oncology, 27*(1), 13–21. https://doi.org/10.1002/pon.4339

Kirk, M. (2008). *Caring for your parents* [film]. WGBH Educational Foundation.

Koerner, A. F., & Fitzpatrick, M. A. (2002). Toward a theory of family communication. *Communication Theory, 12*(1), 70.

Kuang, K., & Wilson, S. R. (2017). A meta-analysis of uncertainty and information management in illness contexts. *Journal of Communication, 67,* 378–401.

Lai, C., Borrelli, B., Ciurluini, P., & Aceto, P. (2017). Sharing information about cancer with one's family is associated with improved quality of life. *Psycho-Oncology, 26*(10), 1569–1575. https://doi.org/10.1002/pon.4334

Laidsaar-Powell, R., Butow, P., Bu, S., Charles, C., Gafni, A., Fisher, A., & Juraskova, I. (2016). Family involvement in cancer treatment decision-making: A qualitative study of patient, family, and clinician attitudes and experiences. *Patient Education & Counseling, 99*(7), 1146–1155. https://doi.org/10.1016/j.pec.2016.01.014

Lamore, K., Montalescot, L., & Untas, A. (2017). Treatment decision-making in chronic diseases: What are the family members' roles, needs and attitudes? A systematic review. *Patient Education & Counseling, 100*(12), 2172–2181. https://doi.org/10.1016/j.pec.2017.08.003

Lau, D. T., Berman, R., Halpern, L., Pickard, A. S., Schrauf, R., & Witt, W. (2010). Exploring factors that influence informal caregiving in medication management for home hospice patients. *Journal of Palliative Medicine, 13*(9), 1085–1090. https://doi.org/10.1089/jpm.2010.0082

Lee, A. A., Piette, J. D., Heisler, M., Janevic, M. R., Langa, K. M., & Rosland, A. M. (2017). Family members' experiences supporting adults with chronic illness: A national survey. *Families, Systems, & Health, 35*(4), 463–473. https://doi.org/10.1037/fsh0000293

Lichtenthal, W. G., & Kissane, D. W. (2008). The management of family conflict in palliative care. *Progress in Palliative Care, 16*(1), 39–45. http://www.ncbi.nlm.nih.gov/pubmed/24027358

Litzelman, K., Kent, E. E., Mollica, M., & Rowland, J. H. (2016). How does caregiver well-being relate to perceived quality of care in patients with cancer? Exploring associations and pathways. *Journal of Clinical Oncology, 34*(29), 3554–3561. https://doi.org/10.1200/JCO.2016.67.3434

Mayahara, M. (2011). Pain medication management by hospice caregivers. *The Journal of Pain, 12*(4 Suppl), P27. https://doi.org/10.1016/j.jpain.2011.02.111

McCarthy, B. (2011). Family members of patients with cancer: What they know, how they know it and what they want to know. *European Journal of Cancer Care 15*(5), 428–441. https://doi.org/10.1016/j.ejon.2010.10.009

McLeod, J., & Chaffee, S. (1973). Interpersonal approaches to communication research. *American Behavioral Scientist, 16*, 469–499.

Meeker, M. A., Finnell, D., & Othman, A. K. (2011). Family caregivers and cancer pain management: A review. *Journal of Family Nursing, 17*(1), 29–60. https://doi.org/10.1177/1074840710396091

Miaskowski, C., Dodd, M. J., West, C., Paul, S. M., Tripathy, D., Koo, P., & Schumacher, K. (2001). Lack of adherence with the analgesic regimen: A significant barrier to effective cancer pain management. *Journal of Clinical Oncology, 19*(23), 4275–4279. http://www.ncbi.nlm.nih.gov/pubmed/11731509

Milberg, A., Wahlberg, R., & Krevers, B. (2014). Patients' sense of support within the family in the palliative care context: What are the influencing factors? *Psycho-Oncology, 23*(12), 1340–1349. https://doi.org/10.1002/pon.3564

Mollerberg, M., Sandgren, A., Swahnberg, K., & Benzein, E. (2017). Familial interaction patterns during the palliative phase of a family member living with cancer. *Journal of Hospice & Palliative Nursing, 19*(1), 67–74.

Nelson, J. E., Hanson, L. C., Keller, K. L., Carson, S. S., Cox, C. E., Tulsky, J. A., . . . Danis, M. (2017). The voice of surrogate decision-makers. Family responses to prognostic information in chronic critical illness. *American Journal of Respiratory and Critical Care Med, 196*(7), 864–872. https://doi.org/10.1164/rccm.201701-0201OC

Nissen, K. G., Trevino, K., Lange, T., & Prigerson, H. G. (2016). Family relationships and psychosocial dysfunction among family caregivers of patients with advanced cancer. *Journal of Pain & Symptom Management, 52*(6), 841–849 e841. https://doi.org/10.1016/j.jpainsymman.2016.07.006

Northouse, L. (2012). Helping patients and their family caregivers cope with cancer. *Oncology Nursing Forum, 39*, 500–506.

Northouse, L. L., Katapodi, M. C., Song, L., Zhang, L., & Mood, D. W. (2010). Interventions with family caregivers of cancer patients: Meta-analysis of randomized trials. *Cancer, 60*(5), 317–339. https://doi.org/10.3322/caac.20081

Olson, D., & Gorall, D. (2003). Circumplex model of marital and family systems. In F. Walsh (Ed.), *Normal family processes* (Vol. 3, pp. 514–547).

Periyakoil, V. S., Neri, E., & Kraemer, H. (2016). Patient-reported barriers to high-quality, end-of-life care: A multiethnic, multilingual, mixed-methods study. *Journal of Palliative Medicine, 19*(4), 373–379. https://doi.org/10.1089/jpm.2015.0403

Peters, J., Dykes, N., Heckel, M., & Ostgathe, C. (2019). A Linguistic model of communication types in palliative medicine: Effects of multidrug-resistant organisms colonization or infection and isolation measures in end of life on family caregivers' knowledge, attitude, and practices. *Journal of Palliative Medicine, 22*(12), 1501–1505. https://doi.org/10.1089/jpm.2019.0027

Pharr, J., Francis, C. D., Terry, C., & Clark, M. C. (2014). Culture, caregiving, and health: Exploring the influence of culture on family caregiver experiences. *ISRN Public Health, 2014*, 689826. https://doi.org/http://dx.doi.org/10.1155/2014/689826

Powers, S. M., & Whitlatch, C. J. (2016). Measuring cultural justifications for caregiving in African American and White caregivers. *Dementia (London), 15*(4), 629–645. https://doi.org/10.1177/1471301214532112

Reigada, C., Pais-Ribeiro, J., Novellas, A., & Gonçalves, E. (2015). The caregiver role in palliative care: A systematic review of the literature. *Health Care Current Reviews, 3*(2), 143. https://doi.org/10.4172/2375-4273.1000143

Ritchie, L., & Fitzpatrick, M. A. (1990). Family communication patterns: Measuring interpersonal perceptions of interpersonal relationships. *Communication Research, 17*, 523–544.

Rodakowski, J., Rocco, P. B., Ortiz, M., Folb, B., Schulz, R., Morton, S. C., . . . James, A. E., III. (2017). Caregiver Integration during discharge planning for older adults to reduce resource use: A metaanalysis. *Journal of the American Geriatric Society, 65*(8), 1748–1755. https://doi.org/10.1111/jgs.14873

Rosland, A. M., Heisler, M., & Piette, J. D. (2012). The impact of family behaviors and communication patterns on chronic illness outcomes: A systematic review. *Journal of Behavioral Medicine, 35*(2), 221–239. https://doi.org/10.1007/s10865-011-9354-4

Roter, D. L., Narayanan, S., Smith, K., Bullman, R., Rausch, P., Wolff, J. L., & Alexander, G. C. (2018). Family caregivers' facilitation of daily adult prescription medication use. *Patient & Education Counseling, 101*(5), 908–916. https://doi.org/10.1016/j.pec.2017.12.018

Schubart, J. R., Reading, J. M., Penrod, J., Stewart, R. R., Sampath, R., Lehmann, L. S., . . . Green, M. J. (2018). Family caregivers' characterization of conversations following an ACP event. *American Journal of Hospice & Palliative Care, 35*(9), 1161–1167. https://doi.org/10.1177/1049909118760302

Schuler, T. A., Zaider, T. I., Li, Y., Hichenberg, S., Masterson, M., & Kissane, D. W. (2014). Typology of perceived family functioning in an American sample of patients with advanced cancer. *Journal of Pain & Symptom Management, 48*(2), 281–288. https://doi.org/10.1016/j.jpainsymman.2013.09.013

Siminoff, L. A., Zyzanski, S. J., Rose, J. H., & Zhang, A. Y. (2008). The cancer communication assessment tool for patients and families (CCAT-PF): A new measure. *Psycho-Oncology, 17*, 1216–1224.

Skinner, H., Steinhauer, P., & Sitarenious, G. (2000). Family assessment measure (FAM) and process model of family functioning. *Journal of Family Theory, 22*, 190–210.

Tallman, K., Greenwald, R., Reidenouer, A., & Pantel, L. (2012). Living with advanced illness: Longitudinal study of patient, family, and caregiver needs. *The Permanente Journal, 16*, 28–35.

U.S. Department of Health and Human Services. (2018). *Quick guide to health literacy: Health literacy and health outcomes.* Retrieved from https://health.gov/communication/literacy/quickguide/factsliteracy.htm

Wang, T., Molassiotis, A., Chung, B. P. M., & Tan, J. Y. (2018). Unmet care needs of advanced cancer patients and their informal caregivers: A systematic review. *BMC Palliative Care, 17*(1), 96. https://doi.org/10.1186/s12904-018-0346-9

Wittenberg, E., Ferrell, B., Goldsmith, J., Ragan, S. L., & Buller, H. (2018). COMFORT[SM] communication for oncology nurses: Program overview and preliminary evaluation of a nationwide train-the-trainer course. *Patient & Education Counseling, 101*(3), 467–474. https://doi.org/10.1016/j.pec.2017.09.012

Wittenberg, E., Ferrell, B., Goldsmith, J., & Ruel, N. H. (2017). Family caregiver communication tool: A new measure for tailoring communication with cancer caregivers. *Psycho-Oncology, 26*(8), 1222–1224. https://doi.org/10.1002/pon.4251

Wittenberg, E., Kravits, K., Goldsmith, J., Ferrell, B., & Fujinami, R. (2017). Validation of a model of family caregiver communication types and related caregiver outcomes. *Palliative & Supportive Care, 15*(1), 3–11. https://doi.org/10.1017/S1478951516000109

Wittenberg-Lyles, E., Demiris, G., Parker Oliver, D., Washington, K., Burt, S., & Shaunfield, S. (2012). Stress variances among informal hospice caregivers. *Qualitative Health Research, 22*(8), 1114–1125. https://doi.org/10.1177/1049732312448543

Wittenberg-Lyles, E., Goldsmith, J., Demiris, G., Oliver, D. P., & Stone, J. (2012). The impact of family communication patterns on hospice family caregivers: A new typology. *Journal of Hospice & Palliative Nursing, 14*(1), 25–33. https://doi.org/10.1097/NJH.0b013e318233114b

Wittenberg-Lyles, E., Goldsmith, J., Oliver, D. P., Demiris, G., & Rankin, A. (2012). Targeting communication interventions to decrease caregiver burden. *Seminars in Oncology Nursing, 28*(4), 262–270. https://doi.org/10.1016/j.soncn.2012.09.009

Wittenberg-Lyles, E., Kruse, R. L., Oliver, D. P., Demiris, G., & Petroski, G. (2014). Exploring the collective hospice caregiving experience. *Journal of Palliative Medicine, 17*(1), 50–55. https://doi.org/10.1089/jpm.2013.0289

Wittenberg-Lyles, E., Washington, K., Demiris, G., Oliver, D. P., & Shaunfield, S. (2014). Understanding social support burden among family caregivers. *Health Communication, 29*(9), 901–910. https://doi.org/10.1080/10410236.2013.815111

Zhang, Y. (2018). Family functioning in the context of an adult family member with illness: A concept analysis. *Journal of Clinical Nursing, 27*(15–16), 3205–3224. https://doi.org/10.1111/jocn.14500

5

The Manager Caregiver

When you are caring for someone and you're bathing them, you're feeding them, you're changing their clothing, you're making sure they're dry, they get to the bathroom, you're helping them. If they've had an accident, you are it. It becomes overwhelming. And it's not that any one thing is hard because it's not. I know how to do those things. It's just that it's so constant. And you're never off. You're on 24/7 and nursing care never is—it's never like that. You have 8 hour shifts, 10 hour shifts, 12 hour shifts, or you can even do 16 hour shifts. But you really can't do it 24/7 without having a break. And I did that for years as his condition got worse and worse and worse. I was getting more and more and more tired.

—Carolina, former nurse, wife of Waldo

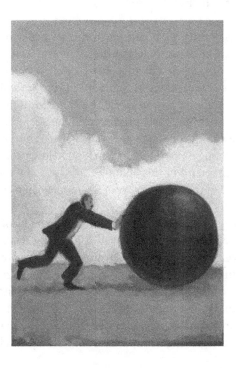

The illustration gracing the first page of this chapter and the subsequent three caregiver chapters are works created by artist Carol Aust. This Manager chapter image can be interpreted as moving an immense weight toward a goal through space and time that has no apparent ending. The person is enforcing their efforts with determination and focus. For the Manager caregiver, the journey of illness is couched in the labors of goal completion and management with many players participating with the Manager serving as governor. If there is movement, then there is care—a significant dimension of the Manager. There is no opportunity to think about things going right or wrong, as the direction and task completion of the caregiver is dominant and the weight of the task immense. It is *what* and *how* they are accomplishing the actions that represent the Manager caregiver. In this illustration, the hazards and pressures of time feel significant and drive the story.

In Chapter 1 of this volume, we describe what the word *chronic* can mean— constant, continuing, ceaseless, unabating, unending. Time does not signal an ending to this kind of illness. Carolina describes this weight so well. We will learn more about Carolina and how she is caring for her husband Waldo. In previous chapters we have shared elements of the story of Maggie. Some of her voice will be interwoven in this chapter in segments that correspond to the overarching themes of the Manager caregiver. Maggie describes the experience of caring for her mom with late stage dementia. Stories from Maggie and Carolina will be central to this chapter, along with additional segments of interviews with other Manager caregivers.

FAMILY COMMUNICATION PATTERNS OF THE MANAGER CAREGIVER

The very core ideas in this book emerge from the theory of family communication pattern, which helps us understand the communication climate inherent in any family structure. From this theory, we have specifically aimed to know about the caregiver existing in one of four patterns in the family communication patterns theory. The communication climate born of those family communication patterns can be named through two primary elements; *conformity* (shared values, attitudes, and beliefs) and *conversation* (what is shared and how frequently it is shared). These two elements each range from high to low, producing four patterns of caregiving (see Chapter 4 of this volume). In describing the Manager for this volume, we now add to the caregiver typology model using concepts initially inspired by Hesse et al. (2017).

The Manager caregiver exists in a communication climate of HIGH conformity and HIGH conversation. The dimension of conformity establishes and protects hierarchies and structures in a family. Harmony and roles are priorities in communication for families with high conformity. The family roles and structures are prioritized above all else in communication. So, the Manager is HIGH conformity, but this conformity can also be classified as WARM. Warm conformity is demonstrated through consistency in upholding rules, sharing beliefs in the direction of equity, designating family times, and valuing family closeness (Hesse et al., 2017). Because of the WARM component to conformity, this caregiver is accustomed to rules about family time together, monitors involvement with family members to remain connected, and communicates family values centered on closeness (Hesse et al., 2017). Putting together the two features, we will describe this caregiver's conformity as HIGH/WARM.

The dimension of conversation is HIGH for the Manager, who experiences frequent and spontaneous conversation among family members. HIGH conversation increases the potential for families to discuss dying, illness, and death and to plan ahead for exigencies of illness. We extend the WARM/COLD description into the dimension of conversation and observe the Manager as experiencing COLD conversation. The priority of the family system to engage readily in interaction may invite readers to assume this is classified as WARM. But the expectation of agreement and assimilation in the conversational topics establish conversation as a COLD theoretical classification. The requirement to express agreement and alignment removes the freedom to include differences and situates the element of conversation as one that can create distance. The group remains cohesive, but they accomplish this in spite of differences that are expected to be suppressed. Putting together the two dimensions of conversation for the Manager, they produce a HIGH/COLD pattern.

The Manager leads care planning and delivery with direct, often swift, and organized action. She is able to communicate readily about the physical and even psychosocial needs of the patient and becomes the center of knowledge for the care. The patient and other family member opinions about health information and decisions are less valued and integrated than for some other caregiver types. The Manager cuts the path of care decisively and other family members support that journey. Becoming an expert on the care recipient is a major focus of the Manager's actions in regard to decision-making, which serves to provide constant oversight but may truncate the care recipients' own personal goals.

Carolina and Waldo each had been married before and began their marriage together when Carolina was 37 and Waldo was 62. Nearly three decades her senior, Waldo had been diagnosed and treated for heart disease (narrowing arteries, arthrosclerosis) but was highly functional as he endured this chronic illness. Then he suffered a massive stroke and subsequently developed vascular dementia that left him unable to walk, talk, or go to the bathroom.

Reflecting current findings about family caregivers and their use of respite care services, Carolina organized supportive home care for small blocks of time to assist her and Waldo. Family caregivers of those living with dementia report the need for respite care as 5.3 times higher than for family caregivers of people with musculoskeletal conditions and 7.7 times higher than for family caregivers of people with cardiovascular or circulatory conditions (Vecchio et al., 2018). Over time, Waldo was impacted more profoundly by these comorbidities and was less and less able to recognize Carolina and their daughter Belle. He required constant care, and Carolina committed to providing that care for him in their own home. Carolina shares details about her own caregiver planning and what she sees as the best approach to care.

The most wonderful thing I can do for Waldo is to make sure that he is comfortable and he's clean and dry and safe at home with us. It's been really good for the family. You know, kids have been able to come and stay and spend time with him. Belle, who lives with us, pops in in the morning and comes in as soon as she comes home from work and says hello to her Dad. The other good thing is that I feel like I am teaching. I put on Facebook what we're doing and why we're doing it and what this journey is. We're doing a great disservice to family members if we have the resources to care for them— what better place to be than at home? And this is how you do it. I will give you instructions, I will help you. I will give you any resource. I have to help you do this [referring to caring for Waldo until death] because it is so worth it. When Waldo is gone, I can look at it. So, I did everything I could for him, and you know that means a lot. He was my knight in shining armor. So, it's really, that's what keeps me going. I am tired. But it's not forever.

For her, remaining in the driver's seat of the care process is not even a decision. It is her duty and an honor. Carolina assesses her approach as the best pathway for caregiving.

MANAGER BEHAVIORS IN THE ILLNESS PROCESS

The onset of illness marks the entry into caregiving. Acute onset is sudden with minimal time for planning or reflection. The Manager acts swiftly, often concealing information to preserve and protect the care recipient and family and maintain conformity. Goal setting and seeking are central points of focus for the Manager, and short-term and immediate goals dominate their activity. This caregiver is a mobilizer of action, which is also evident in gradual onset of illness. In extended onset, the Manager radiates goal setting, but the element of time increases the complexity of the goal planning and the future gaze of this undertaking, with some Manager caregivers taking steps for life after a care receiver dies. Master planning (forward planning goals), positioning (arrange people and things in a particular way), and jockeying (struggle by every means available to achieve something in a skillful manner) emerge in the unfolding of an illness process. The Manager presents to others as *the expert on the care recipient* and performs this role in interactions shared with others. A sense of control and forward movement in the illness process is expressed and enacted by this caregiver. As illness onset continues, the Manager addresses needs that she perceives can be affected such as nutrition, comfort, acquisition of respite care, and providing meaningful experiences for the patient.

In the course of the disease, the Manager may face low- or high-intensity caregiving periods. Whatever the level of intensity, Managers maximize their own activity and maintain hyper vigilance about planning, management, and execution. They arrange whatever elements or moving parts they deem important for the care recipient. As the recipient's needs shift, the Manager rises to the occasion readily to meet the demand by identifying and executing tasks viewed as supportive to the patient. The HIGH/WARM conformity aspect of this caregiver supports their efforts to plan and execute and be surrounded by family agreement and commitment.

Understanding the outcome of the illness can be perceived quite differently across caregiver types. For the Manager, learning about resources and health information is common, but we know that Managers can feel unsure about what they are finding and equally unsure about the best place of care. This caregiver type relies heavily on their own information seeking and swift action, as well as on provider or stakeholder involvement and guidance to further inform understanding, especially as the first source of information. As this caregiver exists in a high conformity family environment, other family members are unlikely to challenge outcome expectations or planning.

The Manager caregiver expresses energy, sometimes effusively; other times, more quietly. But the theme of productivity is present. It may take the form of investment in additional others or literally in the form of producing materials for others to use or enjoy. Idle time is chased away with productivity—in some form. For Carolina, this productivity ranges from sharing medical advice and practical tips for caring to producing personally created crafts.

I want to talk about the equipment that we've had that has helped. We have a three-inch memory foam that does not cause skin to break down. It makes a difference. You don't want a source of infection. It's painful. You just don't want them. And things like a neck pillow that we put around Waldo in bed because as his torso gets weaker; he is listing to one side. So, if you put the neck pillow on, it keeps his neck more upright. The other thing we do is put down a pad in the bed. They are throw away and I put two layers of those because if you have an accident or there's you know, going to be a problem. So that's another trick that we've learned that really works well. There's a lot of tricks that I feel like I can share with somebody that would be in a situation that would make their life easier. With us it's been trial and error. But now we have it perfected.

One thing that has helped is crocheting. The last two years I've made Christmas stockings and pillowcases. I've collected socks and gloves for the homeless shelter. And it's for the LGBT community. These kids are homeless and are 18 to 24 years old. So, this year I made pillowcases and they have bright colors on them for the holidays. I finished that project yesterday [October]. Really, it's a diversion I've also taught one of the caregivers [respite care] to sew with a sewing machine. I am working on two afghans. That's my next push.

Many caregivers demonstrate the quality of vigilance, although the degree of vigilance varies among caregiver types. Managers are sometimes so expert at vigilance that they appear to be at ease with the planning they have executed because it is so detailed, so thorough, and already so complete. So, unlike the common definition of vigilance that may make us think of watching and waiting for threat or danger, the Manager actually takes action to mitigate care needs for the care recipient, but then additionally plans out well in advance and prepares. The Manager can appear to be very put together and in control of the chaos that accompanies chronic illness.

It would be an obvious omission if we didn't point out the Manager's common use of the first-person plural pronouns *we, us,* and *our* that appear readily in descriptions of the caregiving experience. What can at times sound domineering and full of assumption (i.e., speaking for others) is a verbal extension of the commitment to family unity, conformity, and shared goals in place to protect the values and needs of the entire family structure in the face of chronic illness. A HIGH/COLD conversation pattern for the Manager produces a steady stream of information and connection but also an increased level of self-concealment from family members and a willingness to allow the Manager to be the dominant voice and speak on their behalf.

Delegation is a predictable feature in caregiving for the Manager, especially upon patient incapacitation (physical or mental inability to do something). Hands-on delivery of care is distributed to Manager-designated players, including family, friends, and even other healthcare professionals. As incapacitation surges, so does the planning and delegation. Here we share Maggie's perspective on her mom's increasing difficulties and how they can no longer be framed as eccentricities.

In Maggie's Words: Mother's Lying
We really started telling these jokes about our mom being a liar and she would just lie about everything, and we would talk about it comically to make ourselves feel better. Then after Dad died her lying was developing in a new way. One time my Mom told my sister, "yeah, I'm so glad I've never had a drink before." But my dad was an alcoholic and I know my mother drank. I can remember her mixing me a drink when I was a child. Drinking was a big part of our family life when I was young. So now I'm thinking that was an episode, and we just missed it when she said that. My sisters were like, "she just likes to lie." I told my siblings "something is wrong with her. We've got to get help." I'm the sort of person who always wants someone professional to help. So I got a case manager and four of the children got together. I said, "I don't think this is mother lying or being manipulative. She really has something. I think we need to start talking about it."

Some of the stand-out and consistent Manager qualities may demonstrate a lack of inclusion of the care recipient or other family. It's worth underscoring that caregiving is not always met with selflessness and willingness. The cost of caregiving, as we have detailed in this volume, is life altering. So doing the work of caregiving, Manager or not, comes at a high cost to the life of the caregiver. In the wake of nearly a decade of research on the family caregiver types, we are eager to draw a more nuanced picture of the Manager for readers. In early studies of the caregiver, we were able to identify the qualities of dogged researcher and overseer of the care process for a patient (Wittenberg-Lyles, Goldsmith, Oliver, et al., 2012). But it is in the last few years that we have gathered more textured and richer information about this type, which extends the overall knowledge about caregiving and chronic illness.

FAMILY EXPECTATIONS FOR CAREGIVING

For the Manager, a dual emphasis is placed on participatory conversation among family and the obligation to deliver care within existing hierarchical structures of the family system (Wittenberg-Lyles, Goldsmith, Demiris, Oliver et al., 2012). Already-established communication patterns are further cemented for the Manager, and protecting family practices, roles, and expectations is integral to the caregiving this individual undertakes. The Manager is situated as a dominant voice and can seem to act as a spokesperson for the patient and other family members, even serving to quiet other voices in the caregiving effort that may or may not include dissenting ideas (Wittenberg-Lyles, Goldsmith, Parker Oliver, et al., 2012).

> In Maggie's Words: Siblings
> The oldest is my brother Bobby. And then I have Jenny. Nine years older than me. Billy is seven years older than me, and Judith is four years older than me. And I am the baby. We have always protected Billy from things.

This caregiver type is derived from the very best set of motives—the desire to put a plan of action into place with competence and credibility, minimize the difficulty for those impacted by the illness, and offer a stepwise plan to all involved. These are very significant tasks that in most realities are difficult to achieve or achieve in a way that actually eases the burden of illness for the larger family/friend system. For the Manager, family commitment is of the utmost importance in taking a lead on caregiving for a loved one. Family commitment leads directly to family expectations the caregiver perceives, which are resting right under the surface of commitment (see Box 5.1). A common refrain among Managers is that the family is close or the family is central.

Box 5.1

MANAGER DESCRIPTIONS OF FAMILY EXPECTATIONS (2019 DATA COLLECTION)

- *We were raised to be a tight knit family.* (dementia patient, daughter caregiver)
- *I think they're more parents than they are friends, which is different from a lot of people; I see her first as a parent and she sees me first as her son.* (cancer patient, son caregiver)
- *This side of the family is rather large and pretty close.* (COPD patient, granddaughter caregiver)
- *His aunt finally told me, "you just hold this family together."* (Alzheimer's patient, daughter caregiver)

With hierarchical familial roles taking center stage, the honor and duty in performing the work of the caregiver informs the day-to-day living and choices of the Manager. A very high value and judgment is placed on evidence and proof of good care—and this seems to be a personal value and judgment that extends the high conformity family unit for this caregiver type.

Carolina:
I can say at this point, Waldo has never had a bed sore and when a pressure sore was starting, we saw them. We were able to put the barrier cream on it and position him to keep him off of that particular spot.

We believe there are cultural differences among caregivers. This is signified in the data collected by the Family Caregiver Alliance that tells the story of Hispanic caregivers, who give the most time to caregiving, as well as African American caregivers who give the second most amount of time to this labor (Family Caregiver Alliance, 2017) in the United States. Without understanding the specific variables contributing to these trends, we still can see that the pattern of sacrifice for the sake of caregiving is higher among certain populations. In one small study we performed looking specifically at these two minority groups and caregiver types, Hispanic caregivers predominantly were assessed as Managers, while African American participants heavily represented the Partner type (see Chapter 7 of this volume; Goldsmith et al., 2018). But this only creates more curiosity about what cultural factors are at work that might produce these patterns. That there is little known about the many variables compelling certain groups to perform more rather than less caregiving warrants further research.

FAMILY ROLES

The Manager communicates about the news, updates, and plans for care to the patient as well as the family. Information gained, altered, or identified as a result of a meeting with a provider is discussed between the caregiver and care receiver (Wittenberg, Kravits, et al., 2017). Even though Managers seek out health information, their ability to share this information with the patient is not a skill that comes as easily (Wittenberg, Borneman, et al., 2017). The proclivity of Managers to prioritize medical information is not matched with their skills for sharing this information with the patient. There is evidence that the Manager protects the patient from information about their own health to a fault and reports difficulty communicating about matters of illness and caregiving that may seem to threaten family roles and conformity.

In Chapter 1 of this volume, we shared information about goals and how people almost always want more than one thing when they engage in interaction together (Tracy & Coupland, 1990). Because communicators pursue multiple and often competing goals, problems and dilemmas can be common in interaction. Add to this the context of serious illness, and differing goals are quickly compounded. As we have studied this caregiver type, protecting and guiding the care receiver is central to the multiple goals of their caregiving experience. Sometimes these goals are emergent, and sometimes people enter an interaction knowing very clearly what they need/want to achieve, as Carolina explains:

> We are all dying of the same disease. We're doing "now care." And "now care" includes joy, you know? If Waldo is taking lorazepam because he has to have it so he's more comfortable, so he's less combative. Ok. But if you want the gin and tonic, fine.

The core assumptions of communication privacy management theory are that individuals consider themselves owners of their private information and this ownership gives them control of private disclosures (Petronio, 2007). Ownership and control are thus used to navigate the dialectic between disclosure and privacy as individuals have a desire to control private information because of the perceived vulnerability of exposure (Petronio, 2007). Once private information is self-disclosed to another individual, that individual assumes co-ownership of the information. Boundaries are then managed through rule management processes negotiated between individuals (Petronio, 2002). Rule management compels Manager boundaries, and the management of rules seems to be heavily informed by the maintenance of family values and structure. It is easy to draw the connections between protecting some family from health information in accord with family communication climate goals.

In our early observation of Manager caregivers, it seemed that so many of them were in command of medical language. This command created a sense of medical credibility around the Manager (Goldsmith et al., 2016). Speaking with seeming ease about chronic illness and its treatment contributes to the sense of command and action we see in this caregiver type. But we also see some significant command of medical language demonstrated by other caregiver types (in particular the Partner and the Lone). And so it is a reminder of the *assumptions* that we made about this caregiver type that others probably also make about this sort of caregiver—that Manager caregivers have full knowledge, are confident about care decisions, and are equipped with all the information needed to help the care receiver navigate complex care (see examples in Box 5.2). In fact, the Manager caregiver may find they can easily parrot back information due to their extensive focus on seeking health information but may not have a clear understanding of the scope, breadth, and implications of the information obtained.

The family patterns do not create space or opportunity for the Manager to easily share/report caregiving stress within the family, and similarly if there is dissent about care within the family, there is a desire not to disagree or communicate this disagreement about care (Wittenberg, Kravits, et al., 2017). This reality of avoiding dissension is complicated by the significant social support that Managers report experiencing. Surrounded by many who are involved in the unfolding illness of the patient, the Manager is at once upheld by and remains protective of those closest to them.

Box 5.2

Manager Communication Within the Family (2019 Data Collection)

- *It's really just me and my husband and my son in the family meetings, but you know, I just tell them what has gone on during the office visits.* (Alzheimer's patient, daughter-in-law caregiver)
- *I discuss what's going on, what's going to happen next, and if everybody's in agreement with what I'm doing.* (COPD patient, ex-husband caregiver)
- *We really tried to encourage her and lift her up, so it was just fellowship with the family.* (cancer patient, son caregiver)
- *You know you can tell how he's feeling even though he's straight faced most of the time. And my family, everything feels like it kind of gets swept under the rug if it's a big deal. It almost feels a little gossipy, so big information doesn't get out unless it's by word of mouth. So, it feels kind of difficult to talk about medical situations.* (COPD patient, granddaughter caregiver)

FAMILY DECISION-MAKING

In Maggie's Words: She's Not Happy

My mom is not a happy person. She's not happy. She's done. You know, she's still got a long life, but she is done. You know, odds are it's going to be the boys taking care of me [referring to her own sons]. God let's hope they marry nice people. I don't want to live forever. That's not what I value. I try to share sweet happy things I am seeing in mom with my siblings. Like Mother's Day I had my picture taken with her and I shared that picture. The other day mom and I were in the bed. I'll snuggle up with her after she's had her shower. I want them [my siblings] to know that she's declining and if they don't come for another six months, she may not know who they are. Her life now is in the moment. It's me being in the moment with her. I've tried to share a lot of information [with the siblings]. If something happens, I send it out to everybody. Judith didn't do that. So, she still has medical power of attorney. We haven't changed anything. What I've heard is that they'll give priority to the local person they see more. We're fine. I'm friends with her [mother's] physician. We had talked about needing to come up with a little agreement, but Judith has not given us any trouble. She gave us a book with mother's records in it.

Because of the HIGH/WARM nature of the conformity in a Manager's family context, there is a pattern of talking more openly about health issues including death, dying, disease process, side effects, and decisions. Because of pre-existing patterns of connectivity, the illness period that demands caregiving can be perceived as an opportunity to be together and find more ways to connect

(Goldsmith et al., 2015; Melin-Johansson et al., 2012). The harmony pursued by this family type can lead members to seek shared beliefs, values, and accord. But it is important to note that this does not always equate with agreement. And the roles protected in the family can be emphasized over and above conversation and disclosure (Wittenberg-Lyles, Goldsmith, Demiris, Parker Oliver, et al., 2012).

In Maggie's Words: We Want Her

Her hygiene fell apart in that place [assisted living planned by sister Judith]. She was not letting anyone help her with her hygiene. They had horrible challenges with mother's laundry. I know my mom went months sleeping on the same sheets. And she has urinary incontinence. She wouldn't let the housekeepers into her room. Her carpet was filthy. And Judith got the brunt of everything from her. She will always be the middle child. I would say, "Mother you don't smell good. Let's change your underwear." And she would say, "Shut up." Well, that's the worst thing to say to someone. And Judith couldn't take it. She would leave. But it didn't bother me like it did her. I don't worry that my Mother doesn't love me, but Judith does. So I just said to Judith, "we want her here. There's two of us here. She needs more care. She's got to move. We want her. Now it's our turn." We never criticized Judith, but she was not happy. She said, "do not tell mother that this was my idea or that I did not want her." If I lost my relationship with my sister, I have to take care of my mother.

A rigorous medical vocabulary and facility with information related to health is often used by the Manager in healthcare meetings and settings (Goldsmith et al., 2016). This line of conversation is more comfortable for the Manager than for some other caregiver types. As more is learned about the idea of health literacy, we see that language and words really cannot be equated with understanding nor with health behavior (Goldsmith & Terui, 2018). Health literacy is far more complex than the language associated with an illness and its treatment. But it is understandable that the impressions developed by the Manager promote the assumption of high literacy in the use of language, healthcare ideas, and demonstration of adherence to treatment plans (see examples in Box 5.3).

For years we understood the Manager to be the most adept and confident with health information. But other caregiver types in the typology have adeptness equal or even superior to the Manager. We do know that this caregiver is very responsive to information systems, requirements of a healthcare system/setting, and following directions about care, medicine, procedures and side effects with exactness (see Box 5.4) (Wittenberg, Borneman, et al., 2017). Structures and pathways of healthcare provide the Manager with enough architecture to excel in making swift decisions, completing healthcare tasks, and achieving goals of care, no matter how minor they are.

Box 5.3

MANAGERS DESCRIBING MEDICAL ASPECTS OF CARE (2019 DATA COLLECTION)

- *Pills in the tablet form. Oral.* (diabetic patient, granddaughter caregiver)
- *He has vascular dementia and heart failure, and now a GI bleed, comorbidities.* (husband patient, wife caregiver)
- *Encourage them and talking to them. And just trying to give them some feedback of what it can do and what it won't do; it can prolong, you could live longer.* (HIV patient, life partner caregiver)
- *Trying to keep them active with support for everyday activities, like going to the store, shopping up, cooking, trying to keep them as normal as possible and making sure to help them keep on their medication regimen. And get to bed on time.* (HIV patient, life partner caregiver)

Importantly, despite a very competent display of health terms and ease with healthcare concepts, we now know that the Manager's understanding of the healthcare system and determining what information to trust is weaker than that experienced by the three other caregiver types (Wittenberg et al., in review). The Manager relies most heavily on providers for their first source of information (Ferrell & Wittenberg, 2017). Box 5.5 provides some examples.

Respite or home nursing care may be part of the care that some caregivers engage. For Carolina, her description of working with home care staff at once underscores her nursing background and how this informs her caregiving. It also reflects some of the clear patterns of decisiveness and directness that Managers can demonstrate in their relationship/communication with others.

Box 5.4

MANAGER PERCEIVED COMMUNICATION WITH PROVIDERS (2019 DATA COLLECTION)

- *I am a nurse, so I feel like I communicate well with doctors and nurses.* (dementia patient, daughter caregiver)
- *I trust the doctors as far as the medication choices.* (cancer patient, daughter caregiver)
- *We listen to the doctor and then talk it over with the family members.* (cancer patient, close friend caregiver)
- *The doctor chose our current hospital.* (cancer patient, sister caregiver)
- *She gives me the authority to speak for her with the doctor.* (COPD patient, ex-husband caregiver)
- *With doctors and nurses, I am very upfront with them to get what we need.* (cancer patient, sister caregiver)

Box 5.5

MANAGER DESCRIPTIONS ABOUT HOW CARE IS DETERMINED (2019 DATA
COLLECTION)

- *The doctor would tell us to go somewhere if for some reason it was more
  necessary to a different hospital.* (diabetic patient, granddaughter caregiver)
- *Choosing a doctor and a hospital would be my decision. I work at a hospital.*
  (diabetes and Alzheimer's for patient, daughter-in-law caregiver)
- *The doctors there were pretty much how we got the recommendation to her
  doctor.* (cancer patient, daughter caregiver)
- *I prefer the doctor to tell us; I let doctors refer us.* (cancer patient, sister
  caregiver)

Carolina:
I finally wrote down what I expect. I show it to them when they first come.
First day I'll say, this is what I expect. Because most of them are babysitters.
They make sure that they're dry. They make sure that they get fed. But they
don't do the hands-on nursing care of changing diapers, giving a bed bath.
So that level of care, they don't often do. Even though they are supposedly
trained to do that, they may or may not be good at it. It's like one of the
caregivers that we have. I've worked with him, and I said this is the job. Are
you willing to do this? You have to direct these people because they're independent, and they can just sit and read a book. As long as their person is
asleep, that's fine. You know it's too bad that there's laundry in the dryer. And
one thing I tell them is if I'm busier than you, I don't need you. I should never
be busier than you. I tell them, you're here for 10 hours or you're here for four
hours. I'm here for 24 so I will help you turn him. I will help you reposition
him. If he's had diarrhea, I will help you clean him. This is not a problem.
This is my husband. I will do whatever it takes to care for him. But understand that I need a break, and when you're here, this is my precious break.

FAMILY UNCERTAINTY

Illness-related uncertainty has been defined as the inability to determine the
meaning of illness events when these events are ambiguous, highly complex,
lacking information, or when outcomes cannot be predicted. This uncertainty
includes a low degree of confidence in and poor control over various aspects of
life (Karlsson et al., 2014). It is no wonder that uncertainty is a central point of
research in acute, chronic and terminal illness. For some caregivers, working to
maintain uncertainty is actually more comforting than routing out the answers to
uncertainties in the illness journey. But this also calls into question, 'what counts
as something uncertain?' This answer differs for caregivers and for caregiver types.

Practical matters seem to surface for the Manager when it comes to uncertainty. Carolina describes vigilance for the unplanned, and in so doing rectifies the perspective of the Manager, focusing on details, planning and protection.

Carolina:
Even though you have caregivers coming in, they may or may not show up. So, you cannot really leave the person without somebody monitoring . . . you cannot walk away and think that it's going to be okay if you have an agency because it may or may not be. The way I was trained is, you never abandon your patient. You expect that someone you hire to help will be at that same standard [referring to home care or respite care] that you had, but don't ever be fooled that you're going to get that. While I was gone to see my family, the caregivers they had, one of them let Waldo sit in wet clothing from 8:30 in the morning to 2:30 in the afternoon. He did not offer Waldo a urinal. He didn't even know what a urinal was. He had never and didn't ever change him. He didn't walk him to the bathroom. He didn't do anything.

Her words build to a larger description of how uncertainty has led to never trust or believe that there will be help for Waldo without her presence. Uncertainty can exist on a continuum, and our tolerance for it can change over time depending on what the stressors in our life are. Suffering is the partner to uncertainty—both directly connected to the human experience of being in the world and living in the world (Mishler, 1981). Mortal threats to the body and its suffering sets us up to experience uncertainties in the prospect of disease progression, survival, and what life will be like before death.

At first glance, the Manager presents as a caregiver with few health literacy barriers. But research bears out that the Manager reports feeling unsure about where to find the *right* healthcare for the care receiver and is less knowledgeable about the healthcare the patient actually needs (Wittenberg et al., 2019). These are surprising points of knowledge about the most seemingly decisive, credible, and confident caregiver in the typology. But this finding also explains the Manager's reliance on and preference for provider input. Feeling unprepared and without knowledge is something the Manager wants to avoid.

The HIGH/COLD conversation status of a Manager can reduce some uncertainty within the family structure; conversations about the illness and treatment and future plans do take place and establish next steps. But the HIGH/WARM conformity status may truncate some of the conversations that would potentially offer comfort or a lighter load of worry to the Manager---as they so often perform conversational work meant to bring others together and remove uncertainties for the broader circle of support for a care receiver. Communication Privacy Management spells out the boundaries that we draw around information and information sharing with others. This theory paired with the Multiple Goals theory and its explanation about how people create and establish goals combine to explain a lot about uncertainty in caregiving.

CONSIDERING PALLIATIVE CARE COMMUNICATION AND HEALTH LITERACY

Carolina:

So, we went to Houston for like four or five years for care because we felt like we could get better care for Waldo's heart and mind. And it was so hard. So taxing on Waldo. So taxing on me. We couldn't do it anymore. So physically exhausting and, but still, you want to make sure that you didn't miss something. And for every symptom they have everything, you want to treat it. And then at some point in time you have to sit back and say, we've done everything we can. We've done the valve replacement. We've done the AAA [Abdominal Aortic Aneurysm] repair, we've done the leg repair. He's had his cataracts done. We've added medications that will help improve his memory. But your worst nightmare is when you have to throw in the towel and say 'I've done everything. We can't do anymore. This is it. Oh my gosh, we can't do anymore.' So, you have to change your mindset and then go to, what can we do for palliative care? What can we do for comfort? What can we do to create joy in Waldo's life? The life that we have together? And so the nightmare came in that decision of oh, *we've done everything.*

One clear goal of this book is to draw connections for the reader among communication patterns, caregiver burden, and health literacy. Because the Manager is dependent on provider suggestions and information to help shape decisions, there is the great opportunity for the caregiver to experience a caregiving journey that is rescued or even comforted. This caregiver is very responsive to information systems, requirements of a healthcare system/setting, and following directions about care, medicine, procedures and side effects with exactness (Wittenberg, Borneman, et al., 2017). But they remain less sure in their health literacy skills when finding the most appropriate care and the most appropriate providers, despite their facility with the language of disease and treatment. The healthcare professional has many opportunities to collaborate with this receptive caregiver in guiding them toward care that will achieve the best quality of life for the care receiver and caregiver.

Many caregivers in the comforted journey receive both curative and palliative care until the curative treatments negatively impact a patient's/family's quality of life. Carolina describes the experience of integrating the idea that no more curative treatments are going to serve Waldo. The presence of palliative care throughout the disease trajectory ensures far more thorough attention to and protection from suffering for caregiver and care receiver. An awareness of serious and terminal illness is integrated into initial and subsequent discussions about prognosis and care choices in a comforted journey, and we can detect this awareness in the narratives of Carolina and Maggie. Inclusion of the awareness of dying and death heavily impacts shared goals that caregivers/patients and their providers plan and execute, reducing the disillusionment that dominates curative-only treatments for caregivers/patients with terminal diagnoses.

Palliative care establishes (a) shared goals between all medical care providers and their units of care—the patient and family—and (b) the reduction of suffering across all areas of pain (physical, mental, emotional, social) for the patient, caregiver, and family. This goal is simply nonexistent in the isolated journey and is not met until the end of the rescued journey. The comforted journey provides a community of professionals who make the experience of the patient/family their primary concern and transitions patients/families through the stages of care and dying.

Conversely, the rescued journey confronts care receivers and family caregivers who have experienced prolonged suffering with unnecessary treatments in search of a cure and numerous visits with independent healthcare clinicians with no real understanding of the magnitude of their disease; as hospice materializes, the abrupt modification in approach to care may seem brutal, abusive, and disempowering for caregivers who are asked to change their way of thinking about survival. Most things offered in curative and preventative care cease to exist, and all systems are forever changed by the presence of hospice. A curative-only approach to diagnosis augments the willingness of caregivers and care receivers to undergo aggressive care, delaying a hospice referral as well as the patient's understanding of end-of-life care. Despite awareness of the terminal prognosis, some healthcare workers continue to restrict full, open disclosure when working with terminally ill patients and their families (Field & Copp, 1999). Integrating palliative care and hospice into the illness narrative involves a comprehension of terminality, which surfaces from the interrelationship of information, the patient's physical and cognitive decline, and subsequent changes to personality and role (Waldrop et al., 2005). The Manager is heavily integrated into healthcare systems and is responsive to the information and resources provided. As such, structures and pathways of healthcare can provide the Manager with enough architecture to excel in making swift informed decisions, completing healthcare tasks, and achieving goals of care, no matter how minor they are. Similarly, the Manager can engage the shift into noncurative care with the stewardship of healthcare providers and the healthcare system.

SELF-CARE AND THE MANAGER

Although it's not a perfect fit, some aspects of the Myth of Sisyphus are reflected in chronic illness caregiving and in particular, in the experiences of the Managers included in our volume. At the conclusion of a wending Greek epic about Sisyphus, a very wise and prudent person, the gods decided that he would be punished for tricking them. His punishment would last for all eternity. Here was his punishment: Sisyphus would have to push a rock up a mountain; upon reaching the top, the rock would roll down again, and Sisyphus would have to start over. Repeat. Camus, the French philosopher, sees Sisyphus as the absurd hero who lives life to the fullest, hates death, and is condemned to a meaningless task. Camus describes that, as humans, we build our life on the hope for tomorrow, yet tomorrow brings us closer to death (O'Brien, 1961). And that couldn't be more like chronic illness situations. So, the Manager caregiver is working to help the patient maintain not only hope and meaning in this illness experience but also hope and meaning for herself. The freedom for many patients with comorbidities and for their caregivers is no longer found in the bounds of hope for a healthier future, but rather freedom in the immediate present and what those immediate moments offer.

> Carolina: So, we had just gotten him all fixed up, he had just showered. And he had diarrhea. So, we had to take it all down again. What we had just done. And so we had just gotten him fixed up again and he had more diarrhea. And you know, you, if you don't laugh, you're gonna cry. It's exhausting. It's exhausting. And so, you laugh and you, you find the humor in it. You just say, well, you know, why not? Let's just do this again. Why not? This is what we're here for.

To remind us all of the imperative to care for the caregiver, we reiterate the poor health outcomes of the caregiver. Caregivers report intense surges in anxiety, fear, helplessness, depression, anger, guilt, and uncertainty as a result of the unpredictable nature of their situation (Olai et al., 2015). There is now substantive proof that caregivers postpone their own healthcare needs, which helps explain later diagnoses of advanced stage disease in this population (Alliance, 2019).

> Carolina: This is a terrible journey. I feel like jumping out of an airplane, I feel like driving a fast car, you know. It's one of those things where you know you're dealing with death every day and you want to feel. You want to feel the rush. You want to feel alive. And you're tethered to someone's bed and to their needs and you have to put everything that you want and need aside in order to do this.

Depressed caregivers are more likely themselves to have substance abuse or dependence and chronic disease as well. Over a half of caregivers report a chronic condition, nearly twice the rate of non-caregivers (National Alliance for Caregiving, 2018, January). The Manager reports a high need to hide caregiving stress, and this correlates with their high conformity status. Preserving and bolstering the family patterns come at the high cost of concealing caregiver stress and burden away from the care receiver and family system. The Manager reveals confidence and self-efficacy in communication related to social and financial quality of life but suffers in the arena of emotional quality of life (Wittenberg et al., 2019).

> Carolina: Just knowing it's getting closer and closer [Waldo's death], I'm more and more anxious. The doctor has ordered Xanax for me. You know the thing about some of these medications is that sometimes they work and sometimes they don't. And it's gotten to where it doesn't work because I would have anxiety dreams and I'd wake up almost, you know, in panic mode. I thought, I'm better off without it. So then, okay, what's going to help me sleep? You don't want to overdo alcohol either. I don't really go shopping

anymore. I buy things for Waldo online. Things that he needs. But generally, it's been focused on Waldo. What does Waldo need?

This area of burden correlates with the Manager's desire to protect, especially the care recipient, from suffering and loss incurred by chronic illness. A large circle of support is characteristic of this caregiver, but also can help masquerade the Manager's inability to communicate openly in ways that could result in improved self-care. In Carolina's description of her own suffering in the process of unremitting care provision, we see the backstage cost of her labors and her deep desire to find relief. And, in the same breath, she makes it clear she would be nowhere else but with Waldo in their home. She chose over and over to keep him with her there.

Carolina: There was the moment of, well, I'm the memory keeper. The next morning when I walked into Wald's room, he looked at me and smiled in recognition. I knew that he may not know my name, but he knew. So I texted Belle upstairs and she came down and I said, come in and see your dad and watch his face. So you know, she came in and he smiled at her and she kissed him on the check. It was the joy of knowing who she was and the comfort that she was there. And it gave Belle reassurance. And he said to me, are you Palmer? And I said, no. And he said, are you Waldo Ortez? And I said no, that's you. But close. Very very close. And then he called me Honey Bunny, which was one of my nicknames. And I thought, he remembers.

SUMMARY

As the Manager emerges from a communication climate in which there is HIGH/WARM conformity (strong pull to share in similar values, attitudes, beliefs, and familial role expectations) and HIGH/COLD conversation (frequent and restricted communication contacts among the family system), the priority and commitment to family is prioritized. This priority can subvert the needs of this caregiver, and the Manager can find herself protecting the care recipient and, at times, other family members from the challenges associated with understanding a diagnosis and its treatment. The Manager is drawn to professional help and support as well as health information, but this does not mean the Manager is sure about either—and they are strongly reliant on opinions of providers and professionals in their midst.

Because of their facility with the language of treatment and illness, it can be incorrectly assumed that the Manager hasn't accounted for the psychosocial pain for the care receiver. The Manager actually employs similar approaches to all manner of pain (physical, emotional, social, psychological, spiritual) and because of the vigilance of the Manager, the *expert on the patient* is a key-defining trait that is communicated via interactions with providers, family, patient, and other players. This trait positions the Manager to plan and activate care work around and beyond the patient and advance the dynamics of the family system in which they live. Box 5.6 summarizes the Manager caregiver across the topics explored in this chapter.

Box 5.6

Family Communication Pattern
- Conformity—High, Warm
- Conversation—High, Cold
- Caregiver mobilizes others, sets goals, seeks short-term and immediate goals

Behaviors in the Illness Process
- Presents to others as *expert on the care recipient*
- Engages in swift action

Family Expectations for Caregiving
- Leads on caregiving for a loved one

Family Roles
- Communication hub for family, others
- Tendency to conceal information to protect
- Serves as command central for control, action, planning

Family Decision-Making
- Seeks relief through decision-making
- High use of medical language
- Provider is most trusted source of information

Family Uncertainty
- Caregiver presence is necessary to ensure quality care
- Caregiver provides calm and direction in uncertain times
- Reducing uncertainty is a great need

Considerations About Palliative Care Communication and Health Literacy
- Heavily integrated into healthcare systems
- Responsive to the information and resources provided
- Follows directions about care with exactness
- Less confident about finding most appropriate provider
- Less confident about finding best place of care

Self-Care
- Conceals caregiving stress from patient and family
- Copes by filling all time with activity/tasking

REFERENCES

Alliance, F. C. (2019). *Women and caregiving*. Retrieved from https://www.caregiver.org/women-and-caregiving-facts-and-figures

Family Caregiver Alliance. (2017). *Selected long-term care statistics*. Retrieved from https://www.caregiver.org/selected-long-term-care-statistics

Ferrell, B., & Wittenberg, E. (2017). A review of family caregiving intervention trials in oncology. *CA: A Cancer Journal for Clinicians, 67*(4), 318–325. https://doi.org/10.3322/caac.21396

Field, D., & Copp, G. (1999). Communication and awareness about dying in the 1990s. *Palliative Medicine, 13*(6), 459–468.

Goldsmith, J., & Terui, S. (2018). Family oncology caregivers and relational health literacy. *Challenges, 9*(35), 1–10.

Goldsmith, J., Terui, S., Huang, J., Wittenberg, E., & Brockman, K. (2018). Hispanic and African American oncology family caregivers and the Family Caregiver Communication Tool. *Journal of Cancer Education, 33*, S43–S44.

Goldsmith, J., Wittenberg, E., Platt, C. S., Iannarino, N. T., & Reno, J. (2016). Family caregiver communication in oncology: Advancing a typology. *Psycho-Oncology, 25*(4), 463–470. https://doi.org/10.1002/pon.3862

Goldsmith, J., Wittenberg-Lyles, E., & Burchett, M. (2015). When patient becomes caregiver: One couple, two cases of advanced cancer. In M. Brann (Ed.), *Contemporary case studies in health communication* (2nd ed.). Dubuque, IA: Kendall-Hunt.

Hesse, C., Rauscher, E. A., Budesky Goodman, R., & Couvrette, M. A. (2017). Reconceptualizing the role of conformity behaviors in family communication patterns theory. *Journal of Family Communication, 17*(4), 319–337.

Karlsson, M., Friberg, F., Wallengren, C., & Ohlen, J. (2014). Meanings of existential uncertainty for people diagnosed with cancer and receiving palliative treatment: A life-world phenomenological study. *BMC Palliative Care, 13*, 28. https://doi.org/10.1186/1472-684X-13-28

Melin-Johansson, C., Henoch, I., Strang, S., & Browall, M. (2012). Living in the presence of death: An integrative literature review of relatives' important existential concerns when caring for a severely ill family member. *Open Nursing Journal, 6*, 1–12. https://doi.org/10.2174/1874434601206010001

Mishler, E. G. (1981). Viewpoint: Critical perspectives on the biomedical model. In E. G. Mishler, L. R. AmaraSingham, S. T. Hauser, S. D. Liem, R. Osherson, & N. E. Waxler (Eds.), *Social contexts of health, illness and patient care* (pp. 1–22). Cambridge, England: Cambridge University Press.

National Alliance for Caregiving. (2018, January). *From insight to advocacy: Addressing family caregiving as a national public health issue*. Retrieved from http://www.caregiving.org/wp-content/uploads/2018/01/From-Insight-to-Advocacy_2017_FINAL.pdf

O'Brien, J. (1961). Albert Camus, militant. *Columbia University Forum, 4*(1), 12–15.

Olai, L., Borgquist, L., & Svärdsudd, K. (2015). Life situations and the care burden for stroke patients and their informal caregivers in a prospective cohort study. *Upsala Journal of Medical Science, 120*(4), 290–298. https://doi.org/10.3109/03009734.2015.1049388

Petronio, S. (2002). *Boundaries of privacy: Dialectics of disclosure.* New York, NY: State University of New York Press.

Petronio, S. (2007). Translational research endeavors and the practices of communication privacy management. *Journal of Applied Communication Research, 35*(3), 218–222. https://doi.org/10.1080/00909880701422443

Tracy, K., & Coupland, N. (1990). Multiple goals in discourse: An overview of issues. *Journal of Language and Social Psychology, 9*, 1–13.

Vecchio, N., Fitzgerald, J., Radford, K., & Kurrle, S. (2018). Respite service use among caregivers of older people: Comparative analysis of family dementia caregivers with musculoskeletal and circulatory system disorder caregivers. *Aging and Mental Health, 22*(1), 92–99. https://doi.org/10.1080/13607863.2016.1232368

Waldrop, D. P., Kramer, B. J., Skretny, J. A., Milch, R. A., & Finn, W. (2005). Final transitions: Family caregiving at the end of life. *Journal of Palliative Medicine, 8*(3), 623–638. https://doi.org/10.1089/jpm.2005.8.623

Wittenberg, E., Borneman, T., Koczywas, M., Del Ferraro, C., & Ferrell, B. (2017). Cancer communication and family caregiver quality of life. *Behavioral Sciences (Basel), 7*(1), 12. https://doi.org/10.3390/bs7010012

Wittenberg, E., Goldsmith, J. V., & Kerr, A. M. (2019). Variation in health literacy among family caregiver communication types. *Psycho-Oncology, 28*(11), 2181–2187. https://doi.org/10.1002/pon.5204

Wittenberg, E., Kerr, A., & Goldsmith, J. V. (in press). Exploring family caregiver communication difficulties and caregiver quality of life. *American Journal of Hospice and Palliative Medicine.*

Wittenberg, E., Kravits, K., Goldsmith, J., Ferrell, B., & Fujinami, R. (2017). Validation of a model of family caregiver communication types and related caregiver outcomes. *Palliative & Supportive Care, 15*(1), 3–11. https://doi.org/10.1017/S1478951516000109

Wittenberg-Lyles, E., Goldsmith, J., Demiris, G., Parker Oliver, D., & Stone, J. (2012). The impact of family communication patterns on hospice family caregivers: A new typology. *Journal of Hospice & Palliative Nursing, 14*, 25–33. https://doi.org/10.1097/NJH.0b013e318233114b

Wittenberg-Lyles, E., Goldsmith, J., Oliver, D. P., Demiris, G., & Rankin, A. (2012). Targeting communication interventions to decrease caregiver burden. *Seminars in Oncology Nursing, 28*(4), 262–270. https://doi.org/10.1016/j.soncn.2012.09.009

Wittenberg-Lyles, E., Goldsmith, J., Parker Oliver, D., Demiris, G., & Rankin, A. (2012). Targeting communication interventions to decrease caregiver burden. *Seminars in Nursing Oncology, 28*, 262–270.

Spotlight

Existential Crises

A dominant theme in the talk of caregivers, especially those caring for a spouse or the person they most love, is the existential crisis faced when confronted with a terminal or potentially terminal diagnosis in a loved one. Previously held notions about life and death and aging get called into question: Nothing seems certain now.

Lucy, whose husband was diagnosed with Lewy body dementia, describes a world turned upside down. The first year for her was extraordinarily difficult, as she had just had a "big" birthday: problems she had about aging were seriously compounded by her husband's diagnosis. She queries philosophically: If life is all about loss and pain, what's the point? Why are we here? When her husband was first diagnosed, she immediately decided that the couple would have to leave their home: Chuck would have to be institutionalized, and she didn't want to live in their home alone. So she spent the first several weeks searching out a suitable apartment for herself. Later she realized that, although his disease was a progressive one, he might be relatively well and functional for a period of years. But the diagnosis was an upending experience for her.

Quandaries about aging and its concomitant losses, in conjunction with Chuck's diagnosis, plagued her: Can I still do the same things I used to do when I was young, or is my responsibility more to the world, to the universe than to myself? Should I still want to look pretty? Should I start going back to church? Feed the poor? What's the point if it's all about suffering and loss: "It makes you question every single thing in your life." It's no surprise that such questions get called into play when personal crisis is confronted, particularly when a serious health diagnosis is completely unexpected and when it happens to someone relatively young. Yet, Lucy eloquently answers her own existential questions about life's purpose: "I'm hoping that it's not as desolate as I think it is or as sad for a person. I'm hoping there's some spiritual benefit from caring for someone you really, really love, and I hope that compensates for the loneliness that you feel and for the isolation and the sadness—that giving to someone is a compensation. And that I wouldn't know that yet because I haven't been there."

Carolina, aged 63, who has cared for her 92 year old husband for many months, also questions her previous beliefs about aging as she discusses how caregiving has affected her: "It's changed me. First of all, my new motto is live fast, die young, leave a beautiful corpse . . . because old age is not what it's cracked up to be. This is a terrible journey." She wants to ride horses again and engage in more risk-taking activities like jumping out of an airplane in a parachute or driving a fast car. Caregiving for the very elderly makes one question previously held verities: that we all wish to live as long as possible; that we should live life carefully to avoid danger and risk; and that old age offers its own rewards.

Serious chronic diseases and resulting dramatic changes in the patient also bring dramatic changes in the caregiver. Both Lucy and Carolina experience grief, anger, and overwhelming sadness in the course of their caregiving. Lucy asks her therapist: "Will I ever be happy again?" Carolina talks of the anguish of her husband's not recognizing her or their daughter. Yet these caregivers also know profoundly uplifting moments. Lucy says that she and Chuck have never been closer, that they hold hands in bed. And Carolina posts this moving account in Facebook toward the end of Waldo's life:

Last night Waldo had a lucid moment. I sat with him and held his hand. We talked about all the things his hands have done; i.e. caught and played with all kinds of sports balls and rackets, used navigation equipment onboard ship, painted walls and watercolor paintings, held a camera to capture special moments, sculpted, played piano, tied flies for fly fishing, held a scalpel to save limbs and lives, delivered babies and closed eyes of patients whose time to take flight had come, held all kinds of equipment to repair or create, bathed babies, performed magic to entertain and to hold hands of his children, grandchildren, a patient or family member needing reassurance and to hold my hand in marriage. It was a life journey talking about his hands. A lovely moment in time to remember all he has done. A life well lived.

6

The Carrier Caregiver

I'm finding out that Lena's pretty short on temper. A lot of things I think she flies off at the handle. But I think I'm strong. I think I'm dealing with it fine. I think she is probably at the point where she's getting frustrated whenever something is not going right. Just this past week we had a water leak in the house. And then the next morning it was almost like it was my fault that we had a water leak under the foundation. We've had it before. . . . We know the situation. We know it's going to happen. We never know when it's going to happen. But she like came unglued. . . . She said yesterday, she says you know, I enjoy you taking out the trash. I enjoy you doing the dishes now. I enjoy you doing this, but somebody has to take care of me. Somebody has to do things for me. Again, in turn I said well,

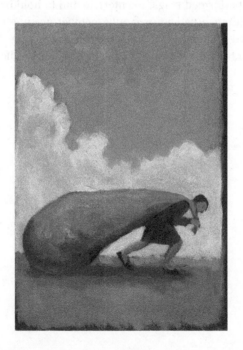

did you call the plumber? She said see? This is what I'm saying. Why don't you just call the plumber? Well, it's something that she's done her whole life, you know. So rather than me asking her again, I just try, I just don't even ask. . . . I don't bring it up.

—Sherman, retired, husband of Lena

This chapter's illustration portrays a person with her nose to the grindstone, hard at work with a focus solely on moving forward. With head down, there is no awareness of the direction in which she is headed, only that it will take hard work to get there. Dedication and loyalty fuel her focus to bear the heavy weight that she carries. Assuming the role of guardian to the family, this illustration represents the Carrier caregiver who shoulders a great deal of pressure. The weight she carries involves responsibility for the family and absorbing the substantial emotional and physical changes experienced by the care recipient. It is enormous and far bigger than any notion of caregiving defined within a healthcare system. With a "be all and do all" approach to caregiving, the Carrier never turns around to see the magnitude of what has been accomplished. Nor does she consider what may lie ahead. Instead she carries on, resolute in her duty and obligation to provide care and demonstrate family commitment. This chapter describes the Carrier caregiver by first explaining the family communication patterns of caregivers like Daniel (and later a return to Sherman) and details the unique attributes of the Carrier in the illness process. This foundation structures an understanding of the family system that gives shape to the communication characteristics of the Carrier caregiver.

FAMILY COMMUNICATION PATTERNS OF THE CARRIER CAREGIVER

Caregiving is considered an opportunity to demonstrate love for the Carrier caregiver, who emerges from a family system with a high conformity and low conversation communication pattern. It is not surprising that the Carrier caregiver focuses on serving as a caregiver, fitting in line with the high conformity pattern from their family. High conformity families prioritize family time together, family harmony, and a structured hierarchical family system. Also grounded in a low conversation family pattern, the solitary role of the Carrier caregiver emerges from a family who does not talk openly about illness and infrequently speaks with each other. The family system functions on the preservation of family through time together rather than time talking together.

It is time together that creates the synergy of family, and this dedication to family time is characterized by a HIGH/COLD conformity pattern. In a HIGH/COLD conformity pattern, family members feel obligated to each other, and mobilization of all family members comes easily. However, in a COLD conformity pattern, it is the Carrier caregiver who self-identifies or is identified by other family members as the family member most obligated to the patient. The caregiving role becomes a primary family functioning tool for the Carrier caregiver who gatekeeps health information and conversation about illness within the family system as a way to keep the family functioning in the midst of illness. By limiting the impact of illness and caregiving tasks to just the caregiver, rather than the family system, the Carrier caregiver is able to preserve family functioning "as is" and protect other family members from the burden of care efforts.

The focus on "doing" in this family and being together allows the family to move forward with decisions and care, despite a low conversation pattern. In a LOW/WARM conversation pattern, there is inconsistency in the topics discussed by family members, ideas between family members are disjointed, and a lack of planned family talk contributes to family disorganization. However, family members may discuss certain topics under specific circumstances allowing some conversations about illness to occur. Yet, the inability and uncertainty of family members to know when it is appropriate and inappropriate for these conversations to occur creates a LOW/WARM conversation pattern. Family members practice self-restraint in sharing their opinions, and nondisclosure functions as a way of honoring the person receiving care. Scheduling time for family conversations to occur can also be difficult for the family to organize. Given the LOW/WARM conversation of the family system, family members may seem aloof, passive, flat, unconcerned, or unresponsive to the patient or other family members because they are unsure about when it is permissible to discuss the illness explicitly. The LOW/WARM conversation climate of the family system makes the Carrier caregiver's ability to make decisions difficult, and conversation among family members consists of raw, unfiltered sharing that creates an intense environment for all parties involved.

CARRIER BEHAVIORS IN THE ILLNESS PROCESS

In contrast to other caregiver types, Carrier caregivers are a steadfast component of the family system, and their role is not influenced by the onset of disease. The first time there is a change in a family member's health, whether it comes severely and intensely through a diagnosis with few symptoms over a brief amount of time (acute) or through a series of symptoms progressing over time (gradual), the behaviors of the Carrier caregiver remain the same. Family mobilization comes easy, requiring little effort to gather all family members to the scene. This is the easy part for the Carrier caregiver who begins to focus on gathering cues about what family members need. The Carrier caregiver presents to others as *the protector of the care recipient* and family in general. As the family comes together to provide support for the care recipient, the Carrier caregiver begins to take stock of what is needed to keep the family functioning. This emphasis on others is complex and prevents the caregiver from being able to delegate. Instead, the Carrier caregiver waits for decisions to be made, by the patient or under the direction of the healthcare team, and this "standing by" approach to decision-making makes it difficult to design a plan for care.

As the length of time for caregiving grows, the Carrier caregiver becomes fixated on the quality of care being provided and responsibilities never change as the caregiver does not delegate. The course of the disease does not impact the behaviors of the Carrier caregiver who remains dutifully focused on the requests of the patient, regardless of disease process becoming progressive (e.g., Alzheimer's disease), relapsing (e.g., multiple sclerosis), or constant (e.g., cancer). It doesn't matter what the diagnosis is, the Carrier caregiver embraces chronic illness with high-intensity caregiving throughout. Evidence of overperformance of the caregiver role is highlighted by Carrier caregivers who work to demonstrate excellent caregiving performance. A majority of family responsibilities are absorbed by the Carrier caregiver who compartmentalizes caregiving and family functioning as separate responsibilities; a piling-on effect begins to build overtime as there is limited outsourcing of caregiving responsibilities within and outside of the family system.

Understanding and discussing the outcome of the disease is not considered by the Carrier caregiver to be their responsibility. Discussing the illness has been thought about carefully by the Carrier caregiver and is viewed as something that must be initiated by the patient. Consonant with a LOW/WARM conversation pattern, this caregiver waits for the patient to decide if he or she wants to talk about the illness or make decisions about the future. The patient is expected to lead these discussions, and if the patient does not initiate the discussion, the Carrier caregiver feels it would be inappropriate and disrespectful to force the patient to talk about these difficult topics. This caregiver doesn't reference the illness and communicates with the patient in a limited, "small-picture" way, often suppressing difficult decision-making discussions with the patient. Acceptance of illness and treatment choices can be confounding because of limited talk. This caregiver type is most likely to acquiesce to other family members for discussions about the illness.

Regardless of the degree to which the patient requires support for routine activities, ranging from everyday support for eating, bathing, toileting to providing medication oversight and transportation to medical appointments, the Carrier caregiver is prepared to do it all. These caregivers overperform their role in the family structure to avoid stressful discussions and minimize illness impact on the patient as well as on other individuals in the family. The Carrier caregiver goes outside the family to process burden or find relief as it is not considered appropriate to discuss within the family. Motivated by an obligation to do things for family members, the Carrier caregiver is acutely aware of family expectations for caregiving.

FAMILY EXPECTATIONS FOR CAREGIVING

Within the Carrier's family system, illness is considered a private family experience. It is not only a private experience for the family in a way that should exclude others from assisting and participating, but it is also a private experience not talked about within the family. LOW/WARM conversation patterns about illness and HIGH/COLD conformity produce implied, high-pressure family expectations for their role as caregiver, which are commonly steeped in cultural beliefs, values, and obligations. Almost automatically, with little thought or consideration of any other alternative, the Carrier caregiver assumes the caregiving role and perceives their role as essential to continued family functioning.

Daniel

I have been a caregiver to my grandmother since I was 17, I am now 27, so about ten years [of caregiving]. My grandmother took care of me since I was a baby so when she started getting older, even before the cancer I was her caretaker. I felt like I owed it to her and of course because I love her very much. I'm Mexican and from a very young age we learn to always respect our elders, and care for them when they can no longer care for themselves.

The Carrier caregiver perceives the caregiving role as part of their obligation to family, established either culturally or socially. Daniel's family is not unlike many Mexican American families where care is provided to multiple family members simultaneously by one family member or successively to several family members by one family member (Evans et al., 2017). High conformity is based on cultural background, which dictates appropriate and expected roles for caregiving and a sense of duty to provide care and support and help for the elderly, especially parents. Among Asian American, Hispanic American, and African American caregivers, the role as caregiver is an expected part of life passed down from generation to generation (Lee et al., 2018; Pharr et al., 2014).

A deep commitment to reciprocity motivates the Carrier caregiver who feels that they owe it to the care recipient to provide quality patient care (Evans et al., 2017). For Daniel, care received as a child motivates him to provide care to his grandma. The commitment to reciprocity is also felt by his grandma who engages in direct talk about care:

My grandmother's diagnosis is stage two non-small cell lung cancer; it was stage one but it is spreading. She got it after years of smoking. When she was diagnosed I forced her to quit which was a battle to say the least. . . . In the beginning when my grandmother first got cancer, she just thanked me for taking care of her but that she would not be a burden for too long.

Open conversation about daily living and its impact on health are permissible, as a way of conveying love and support for the ill family member. Daniel is able to candidly address his grandma's smoking, and with the diagnosis, his grandma is able to convey thanks for his care. These two topics are permissible in the family system around the topic of illness. They acknowledge family commitment to serve and care for elders and the appreciation elders have for that role.

Carrier caregivers are often recognized as the caregiver within the family, and several reasons account for this: a prior commitment to provide the care (e.g., marriage), the caregiver is considered most available because their occupation does not require work outside of the home and is thus more available and flexible, they do not have much of a social life, they are the healthiest in the family, or the caregiver needs a place to stay and it works out for them to be the caregiver (Evans et al., 2017). Although daughters are highly susceptible to the Carrier caregiving role, in Daniel's family he is recognized as best suited for his grandma's care:

> It's tough because I feel like I'm the one that has to do a lot of the work, because a lot of the family members have other obligations like family and kids, etc., I'm the one that's a single student so it's like I have to do a lot of the care taking myself. I do have other obligations but it's not as big as the other family members.

It is easy for the Carrier to accept the family's unspoken rationale for their role as caregiver because they believe that their role as caregiver is a vital contribution to the well-being of family. Early expectations about caregiver responsiveness and reliability are learned within the family system and are carried into adulthood (Dark-Freudeman et al., 2016).

For the Carrier, the bar for quality caregiving is set by a deep obligation to family. The only measure of success is the quality of their care and the opinion of family members, especially the care recipient. This caregiver's goal is to work hard to meet family expectations, and family obligation influences the commitment to provide care (Paulson & Bassett, 2016):

> She was expecting to die soon after her diagnosis but it's been over a year and she's still fighting. . . . At first, she had no fight in her, she just wanted to let the cancer play out. When she told me this obviously I was devastated, I mean this was the woman who helped raise me. But, it made me want to be a better caregiver to make her as comfortable as possible in this difficult and painful time in her life.

The drive to do all caregiving tasks themselves and be "a better caregiver" informs the Carrier's perceived expectations for caregiving as a duty and responsibility to be selflessly carried out.

FAMILY ROLES

Chronic illness impacts all facets of family life. Carrier family systems accomplish quality caregiving without directly making care decisions and with little conversation between caregiver and care recipient (Wittenberg-Lyles et al., 2012). Vitally important to the Carrier caregiver is to carry out the requests of the care recipient, yet communication about illness is inferred through the activities of the caregiver. The relationship between Carrier caregiver and patient is top–down, with the care recipient leading care decisions and the caregiver's goal being to focus on permissible topics of conversation and carry out decisions. Although communication within the family is supportive and other family members are there to assist with supporting patient care, the Carrier caregiver prefers to take on caregiving on behalf of the family.

Sherman

> I feel like my mind is in a hundred different places . . . [my wife] does all that secretarial stuff. She's been a secretary her whole life. So, I rely on her to take care of my business, my personal life, and everything. . . . If I was a computer guy, I could go online and use some, take away some of the billing for her, do some of that stuff. But I have never done that in my 70 years, and it's nothing easy that I could just jump in and do.

Similar to Daniel, Sherman is a Carrier caregiver and experiences the change that is forced upon families when a chronic illness such as cancer is diagnosed. Sherman and his wife Lena have been married for 48 years and have one daughter and three grandchildren. Last month Lena was undergoing pre-operative tests for an upcoming surgery when a lesion was identified on her lung. She was later diagnosed with stage III lung cancer and started initial treatment within the last 30 days. Feeling indebted to Lena who has ran the business side of his dental impression practice, as well as their family home, Sherman naturally steps into place as her caregiver. Sherman's caregiving role is inferred within the family system because he is the spouse and because he can physically do it ("I don't take a pill for anything, and I'm 72 years old. I think I'm pretty healthy.).

Unlike the Manager carrier who is a master delegator, the Carrier's role within the family becomes the solitary role of caregiver. Additional family roles and their unique family identity are lost for the Carrier. These caregivers throw themselves into caregiving by abandoning all of their own personal pleasures, attempt to assume family roles for the care recipient, and have a hard time asking for caregiving help themselves:

> I gave up riding my motorcycle. I gave up my antique cars. I gave up everything to devote to her, and it's hard for me to ask my daughter to do anything. My daughter is always asking her [his wife] to do something, and I'm always available to take the grandkids to the hockey, soccer games or practice, and do all that.

Sherman feels obligated to provide dedicated, concentrated attention to his caregiving role and abandons his own sense of self to accomplish this. The compounding stress for the Carrier caregiver is the imbalance of family roles as they attempt to take on tasks for the care recipient and try to establish a new family pattern that protects the care recipient from family responsibilities. The emphasis on protection is justified by a self-proclaimed open family system:

> We're a close family. We're a close family, even though it just was the three of us for years. . . . We don't keep any secrets, and we tell each other, you know, what's on our mind and what's going on with the family.

Communication within the family is tight but includes a LOW/WARM conversation pattern. The Carrier's definition and description of a close family is about commitment to family obligation rather than communication about illness. In Sherman's family, his wife's elderly mother has not been told about her cancer diagnosis. Sheltering other family members is acceptable and viewed as necessary within the family. Especially among dementia caregivers whose caregiving role is often longest in duration, there is sustained commitment to the relationship by protecting the identity of the person with dementia (Roberto et al., 2019).

The goal of protection also motivates new and different ways for the Carrier to talk about the illness, and this leads to limited communication with the care recipient. On one hand, the Carrier reports an open communication pattern and a close relationship with the care recipient, as Sherman explains:

> I think she's pretty open to speak about anything and everything . . . personal things we talk about . . . family we talk about. I can't think of anything that she would say "No, I don't want to talk about that or I could never hear." I've never heard her say anything like that.

However, the Carrier's role in communication with the care recipient is limited because the Carrier is hesitant to discuss any concrete topics related to the illness. Sherman continues:

> Communicating with my wife is most difficult because I don't want to hurt her feelings, and I don't want to, at this point in our life, I don't want to upset her in any way. I don't want to make it harder on her with what she's going through right now.

This contrast between a perceived open communication pattern and the difficulty of discussing illness is felt by Sherman who wants to maintain closeness with his wife. Because this closeness is dependent upon feelings of family commitment, illness can present an uncertainty that causes high topic avoidance and lower levels of perceived social support (Dark-Freudeman et al., 2016). Like most Carrier caregivers, Sherman has the utmost concern for his wife's feelings and does not want to jeopardize the closeness he feels with her by bringing up uncomfortable topics.

As a result, the Carrier caregiver concentrates on letting the care recipient be the driver of illness discussions, honoring the LOW/WARM conversation pattern, and this family role includes avoiding potentially emotional discussions about illness:

> I think even last night she woke up in the middle of the night. She had a cramp in her leg, and she said oh, "what do I have to look forward to, you know?" I think, to be honest with you, I think I'm okay with it. I kind of turn the other ear and I don't start any kind of argument. I just listen to her vent. And, I think I'm okay. . . . She's just really short when it comes to her temper right now, so nothing can be going right. Before she was able to cope with a lot of things, but now she's just a little bit more frustrated. . . . At times she'll just clam up, and then I get a one-word answer. . . . I think at some point she's probably a little scared, which we all are, of course. . . . I think basically she's the one that has to make a decision.

Sherman is aware that his wife is processing the magnitude of her illness and the changes it brings; however, he does not address it openly. Nor does he tell his wife that he is also afraid of what the future will bring. Instead, he "lets her vent" and perceives that this silence about her illness brings her comfort and support. While relationship quality reduces the negative impact of caregiving and increases satisfaction with the caregiving role (Aloweni et al., 2019), this does not mean that open communication is occurring.

Carrier caregivers typically report that they discuss fears about treatment or dying with the care recipient (Wittenberg et al., 2017); however, these conversations are not characterized by an exchange of emotions, feelings, and values.

The Carrier caregiver's family role includes the invisible work of sounding board for the care recipient who experiences adjustments to life, loss, and feelings of mortality. Carriers perceive that this is a natural part of their caregiving role and that this occurs because of the closeness with the care recipient and their own personal strength to bear witness:

> Right now, when she says something, I say to myself well, I know she's stressed. I know she's under . . . the feeling that she has no control over. If she does have control, uh, what am I looking for? Um, just, just her, she's not comfortable in her, in her body right now. She, her mind is, is picking on me. Because I don't see her that way when I'm around the family. It's only me if she knows she can say that and get away with, you know. I just kind of shrug my shoulders and put my arm around her. And I say we'll get through this. We'll get through this. I think at certain times I don't think she wants to give up. But I think she just feels that she's being picked on and why is somebody up above doing this to me.

Sherman is compassionate about Lena's agitation and that it manifests in their relationship, and he considers this part of the caregiving role. For Carrier caregivers, caregiving is considered a moral and cultural duty that increases their willingness to serve and is believed to enhance relationships within the family (Zhang et al., 2019). Within the Carrier family system, this closeness is enhanced by not talking directly about illness; here, Sherman acknowledges Lena's feelings by emphasizing that they will get through the illness.

The commitment to family privacy also means that the Carrier perceives that their family role is to keep the illness experience and caregiving responsibilities private. Embedded in this scope of caregiving is also the belief that the care recipient's thoughts and personal coping processes are private. The Carrier does not share with others how the care recipient is doing psychosocially. These caregivers perceive that this is necessary for ensuring family cohesion. For Daniel, dedication to *la familia* shifts the focus from the stress of caregiving to the Carrier's focus on the gains of caregiving and reluctance to admit burden (Evans et al., 2017).

When families have difficulty sharing emotions and processing emotions together, greater distress occurs (Dark-Freudeman et al., 2016). The Carrier caregiver is aware of this and works to minimize stress in other family members by avoiding talk about the illness, not seeking support, and relying solely on themselves to manage distress (Dark-Freudeman et al., 2016). When asked if he would like help, such as talking with a social worker, Sherman replied:

> I don't think I need anybody to vent to. I think I'm really okay with it, accepting the way she is now and accepting, she's more the boss now is what I'm trying to say. Maybe because, she's always done everything for me, and now it's . . . I should step up and do a little bit more. . . . I would be very open to that [talking one-on-one with a social worker], but I think at this point I think I have, I think I'm in control. . . . I think I'm in control of myself is what I'm saying. I feel strong about it.

As most Carriers feel that caregiving is owed to the care recipient, they remain steadfastly loyal to this family duty and hide caregiving stress to prioritize family cohesion and functioning (Wittenberg et al., 2017). Just as Sherman explains, the Carrier caregiver commonly feels in control of caregiving as they have not yet addressed the emotional or psychosocial ramifications of the illness within their family. Processing burden and finding relief typically comes from outside the family for the Carrier as an important part of their family function is exhibiting the strength to carry out the expected caregiving role.

FAMILY DECISION-MAKING

Carrier caregivers perceive that their role in decision-making is to accommodate the care recipient and other family members and follow the directions of the healthcare team, especially the physician. During family meetings, the Carrier is an active contributor who focuses on physical care tasks and medication regimens. The Carrier caregiver is keen on knowing the services, roles, and hierarchies of healthcare contexts, as the family is not integrated into decision-making and information finding (Wittenberg et al., 2019). They enjoy quality relationships with healthcare providers as they actively work to communicate and learn more information about their job as caregiver.

The Carrier caregiver has a small role in the decision-making about treatment and care. Decisions are predominantly made between the patient and healthcare team, with a small degree of caregiver influence (Laidsaar-Powell et al., 2017). There is heavy reliance on the physician and healthcare team for decision-making. Daniel describes his role when meeting with the healthcare team:

> We found out the cancer spread and we met to discuss where to go from there. I stayed quiet and really took the information the doctor was saying, trying to figure it all out and process it. Nothing really happened after the meeting except my grandma asked me and only me really what she should do. I stayed pretty quiet only asking the doctor questions personally after the meeting was over, one on one.

Daniel describes his role as supplemental to his grandma, and he focuses on learning more from the doctor. The Carrier caregiver looks to the care recipient to make decisions about care. Carrier caregivers do not perceive that their role is anything more than "doing" and would never impose their own opinion. Daniel describes that the most important aspect of his role is to make sure that his grandma gets the care she wants:

> I trust the doctor but when the cancer spread I tried to take my grandmother to another doctor but she refused. She wanted to stay where she was already comfortable and I respect her decisions. I let my grandmother choose her treatment, but she usually chooses what the doctor recommends is best and I agree with that.

Overall, family decision-making does not happen because illness is often kept private between the care recipient and the caregiver (Goldsmith et al., 2015). Although Daniel's mom and her sisters are local family, decisions are primarily made between Daniel and his grandma ("My grandma asked me and only me"). Conflict only occurs for the Carrier caregiver when the care recipient is unwilling to assume authority in making their own care decisions (Benson et al., 2019). A lack of involvement of other family members is often the preferred position for the Carrier caregiver who doesn't want other family members to be impacted by care responsibilities and because there is high value placed on the "private" relationship with the care recipient.

In addition to feeling obligated to the care recipient, Carrier caregivers also have a sense of obligation to the physician and have a strong preference for paternalistic communication. In a paternalistic physician–caregiver relationship, the physician is recognized as the prototypical parent figure, assumed to be working with the best of intentions. Similar to the Carrier's feelings of obligation to family, the paternalistic pattern focuses on obligations with the implication of trust between physician and patient (Eliassen, 2016). Daniel feels this way:

> I have a lot of respect for my grandmother and I treat her with respect as well. As far as the doctors and nurses I am very appreciative of them and the hard work they do and I trust that they always have the best intentions.

Older adults, like Daniel's grandma, can be reluctant to question medical authority, and the Carrier is similarly reluctant to challenge the care recipient's autonomy; this is often deeply rooted in cultural beliefs (Roeland et al., 2014). For example, the Chinese culture emphasizes both strong cultural beliefs about caregiving expectations and well as traditional roles within families. Among Chinese women, respectfulness is an accommodation style used by women who have a high sense of family obligation (Wiebe et al., 2018). Cultural factors result in a limited desire or ability to participate in treatment decision-making, misunderstanding of disease, less desire/need for information, inaccurate assessment of risk, and fewer questions asked of healthcare providers (Campesino et al., 2012; Costas-Muniz et al., 2013; Mead et al., 2013).

When communicating with physicians, Carrier caregivers have difficulty asking questions about the future and avoid conversations about pain and symptoms. Instead, the Carrier keeps the focus on preventive care, physical care, and things within the scope of caregiving. Here's one caregiver's summary of a recent family meeting prompted by the patient's pain:

> We were addressing the fact that her pain wasn't, has not been resolved. So, we did meet with her internist and the pain management team and they devised a new therapy and added aqua therapy to her treatment. My opinion was that she needed more physical activity and aqua was recommended.

This Carrier caregiver does not express concern over the patient's pain but rather focuses on the needed remedy. No discussion or elaboration about the patient's pain occurs and there is no exploration of other psychosocial factors that could be causing pain. The Carrier caregiver finds comfort in addressing physical care and medication management topics. Since conversations about the future of the illness are difficult between the care recipient and caregiver, there is typically no paperwork such as an advanced directive or living will available. In Daniel's case, his grandma had no living will despite having an advanced cancer diagnosis.

FAMILY UNCERTAINTY

While all caregivers have high uncertainty, especially as the illness journey begins, the Carrier caregiver has the highest uncertainty in feeling prepared (Wittenberg et al., 2017). Family conformity about the role and expectations of the family caregiver are understood; however, inconsistency in what can be discussed among family members in terms of the illness creates uncertainty for the Carrier. There is little room for discussing caregiving within the family system, yet Carrier caregivers are eager to prove their ability to provide quality care and seek recognition and value for their role.

Worry about caregiving performance is the Carrier caregiver's expression of uncertainty. Worry about caregiving has to do with the caregiver's self-appraisal of their caregiving performance which influences caregiver well-being (Heyzer et al., 2019). Concern for their ability to do more and do better is prominent among Carrier caregivers and can be caused by feelings of self-criticism and guilt. This is especially salient among collectivistic cultures, such as Asian communities, where obligation values caring for family members (Lim et al., 2014). Among Chinese adult children, an emotionally close relationship with the parent being cared for increases worry about caregiving performance (Liu & Bern-Klug, 2016). Research with Chinese families who have a high respect for parents culturally has found that a stronger sense of family obligation lowers emotional, social, and physical burdens (Guo et al., 2019; Lee et al., 2018). However, the degree to which the caregiver feels attached to the care recipient as well as a weaker sense of family obligation may lead caregivers to feel unprepared for caregiving (Paulson & Bassett, 2016).

Spousal caregivers are also likely to feel that they can do better, as this Carrier caregiver describes:

> I wrote down everything he had for lunch. I would find out what he had for lunch, what he had for dinner. I would add up the calories and I would call the dietician there and tell her, this is what he had today. He's still losing weight. What can we do, how can I make every calorie count? How, what can I do? And, it was probably a couple times a week I was on the phone calling, wanting information—what can you tell me to do? This is what I'm doing, now tell me what I can do more. And then it never seemed to be enough. But it was, again, he wouldn't drink Ensure for a long time; his tastes changed, there was almost nothing that he would eat, so that was another challenge. So, diet issues were big challenges.

This Carrier caregiver felt that her husband's inability to gain weight had to do with the success or failure of her caregiving. She describes two challenges related to "diet issues"—trying to get a lot of calories into her husband's diet when he was eating and later trying to get him to eat. Both of these were out of her control but became her focused element of caregiving. This Carrier caregiver goes on to describe how her whole life revolved around her caregiving role:

> I have wonderful parents, but they live about twenty minutes away. It's not too far, but there were times that I needed a distraction, even if it was for them to come over and my husband would be sick and lay in bed. They would come

and sit with me, and we would just talk. So that was what I needed. I needed visitors as a distraction to keep my mind from seeking what needed to be done next. I was trying to look ahead always, to see what I could do next.

Carrier caregivers always feel like they should be doing more and always prepare to be "on duty" for any caregiving needs. This proclivity to be concerned with caregiving keeps them from initiating any self-care.

Rather than turning to healthcare team members to learn more about the long-term impact and ramification of disease, the Carrier caregiver uses this time to report on caregiving challenges and seeks confirmation from providers to reduce uncertainty about caregiving. Throughout the duration of care, the Carrier maintains a "small picture" perspective of the illness by focusing on daily care tasks and challenges and has difficulty seeing any long-term implications. The complete perspective of the illness duration becomes a challenge for the Carrier caregiver who focuses on small details that do not reveal the entire story of the disease trajectory. Food and nutrition are examples of the small details in illness care that are important to the Carrier, as described in the following:

> There was a time when it was very hard for my husband to eat. . . . I would take a peach slice, just from a can, a small peach slice, and it would take him an hour to eat that peach slice. . . . He wouldn't just take the slice. I would have to cut it in half and then he said, cut it in half again. So, I would have to force that. And he wanted it in equal portions. I mean, it was that particular on how he would have to eat that, each slice. And he, and, so there was a time whenever I, I did ask him, well what can I, what can I fix you to eat? And he just said, well, I just don't know. And I said, well, when you don't know, I do. So, I fixed something.

Caregiving challenges are opportunities to be a better caregiver for the Carrier who takes pride in finding solutions to caregiving quandaries. With caregiving connected to family obligation, the Carrier caregiver has great psychological endurance and can instill a sense of reward through caregiving (Roberto et al., 2019).

The need for recognition for a job well done is desired by Carrier caregivers—not from family members but from healthcare providers who are considered the ultimate authority on quality care. This caregiver type does not desire tangible, instrumental support; rather, they desire acknowledgment and emotional support (Benson et al., 2019). Carriers have a high need for accolades to bolster their confidence and feel valued for their efforts, as detailed here in a caregiver's memorable moment:

> I remember to this day was when I was with my mom at the doctor's clinic for a general checkup . . . my mom, she's just grumpy all the time. Sometimes she's a hassle to take care of, but I love that woman. A nurse saw that I was taking care of my mom and she said "You have very good patience and that's what makes a good caregiver, a great caregiver, because you're always constantly taking care of them. You have patience for the person and that's what we're supposed to do. I've

seen some caregivers who treat the patient or the person they're taking care of like they are not a person." ... And honestly, my mom has type 2 diabetes ... [she is] suffering so I don't want to be another reason for her to suffer even more. I really took those words at heart. ... It made me feel great honestly because it was a compliment and I rarely get any of those. So then when she told me, "You know what you're actually a pretty good caregiver," it just gave me a boost to my self-esteem to continue. It's those small details that really make a difference at the end. Maybe to her it was just like some random words that she'd just put together at the time of the moment, but those words really stuck with me.

Comments from healthcare providers—in this case, a nurse—are especially important to the Carrier as this is often missing from the family system. Although there is a need for emotional support and recognition for their commitment to family care from other family members, a LOW/WARM conversation pattern means that family members do not know when or how to give such accolades. As a result, there is often little confirmation or validation of the Carrier's performance within the family system despite high family expectations. Daniel describes this:

It is hard being the main caregiver because whenever anything happens it is my fault because according to them I wasn't taking care of her. I get frustrated all the time but I hide it. All because I do not want my grandma to see me angry and have her think she is some sort of burden. Everyone has something to say about the way I care for my grandmother but I don't see them doing a better job or anything at all.

Carrier caregivers do not feel resentment at family members for lack of instrumental support but do desire emotional support. Rather, the Carrier caregiver has a propensity to be fully self-aware and accept unresolvable conflicts (Benson et al., 2019). Rationalizing that this is best for his grandma, Daniel hides this stress about a lack of family support and chooses not to address it with other family members. This is one way he prioritizes family harmony over his own needs.

CONSIDERING PALLIATIVE CARE COMMUNICATION AND HEALTH LITERACY

The Carrier caregiver is motivated to protect: to protect the care recipient, to protect other family members, and to protect the family by keeping the illness private and within the family system. Family expectations for caregiving are often culturally or socially specific for the Carrier, with care expected between spouses and for elders commonly fueled by feelings of indebtedness or obligation. For family members, the Carrier caregiver is the natural choice for the role, and this role becomes the focus of their daily life. The emphasis on privacy sets both the Carrier and care recipient on an isolated illness journey where conversations about illness focus solely on cure-only and restorative care. This supports the communication pattern established in the family and the beliefs about caregiving held by the Carrier caregiver. While there are huge family expectations for caregiving, there is also little internal family acknowledgment. Carriers worry about caregiving performance and look to healthcare providers for validation and recognition of their caregiving role. The isolated journey is fortified when healthcare providers focus only on the Carrier caregiver's success in caregiving.

However, Carrier caregivers maintain a very close hands-on approach to caregiving, insisting that caregiver tasks are performed by them and them alone (HIGH/COLD conformity). Given this role in care, the Carrier caregiver has a close connection and acute awareness of the physical and emotional changes taking place with the care recipient; however, LOW/WARM conversation patterns create an uncertain environment for sharing this awareness and the feelings associated with these changes. As change continues to occur and the course of disease moves forward, the introduction of hospice by healthcare providers will trigger a rescued journey that asks families to change this pattern and to begin sharing feelings. Thus, the care experience feels like a "rescue" because the Carrier caregiver has been well aware of these changes, has suppressed these feelings, and is now given permission to share these thoughts and emotions. The entry of hospice in the rescued journey for the Carrier caregiver provides the clear okay to discuss illness in the family. Prior to this the family experienced a "yellow light" approach where discussions about illness were risky. Hospice enters in the rescue journey and encourages and promotes discussions about illness. The hardest part of the rescue for the Carrier caregiver is the HIGH/COLD conformity pattern, which emphasizes privacy. Privacy is important to the Carrier caregiver, and family decision-making does not take place as care decisions are considered the responsibility of the care recipient and the healthcare team. Thus, with the Carrier caregiver, patient privacy and dignity need to be emphasized and reassured for the rescued journey to occur.

The comforted journey for the Carrier caregiver requires palliative care communication that recognizes the shared illness experience between the caregiver and care recipient. The HIGH/COLD conformity pattern that emphasizes family obligation drives Carrier caregivers to fixate on physical caregiving, allowing them to postpone the threat of change to the family system. As a result, they may experience separation anxiety as part of anticipatory grieving, making discussions about palliative care or end-of-life care difficult (Coelho et al., 2019). Given the LOW/WARM conversation pattern that has limited communication between caregiver and care recipient, the Carrier caregiver is likely to experience previous relational failures and loss of expectations of affection, which contributes to difficulty in making decisions about unmet needs (Coelho et al., 2019). The comforted journey must include communication that emphasizes palliative care as an opportunity to strengthen the caregiver–care recipient relationship, thereby developing a meaningful and hopeful experience. Engaging in palliative care communication that emphasizes the close relationship resulting from the shared illness experience will help the Carrier caregiver to find a comforted illness journey characterized by open awareness and the productive experiences of illness.

Worry about caregiving performance motivates information seeking; however, Carrier caregivers limit their information-seeking behaviors in an effort to manage uncertainty. This does not mean that Carrier caregivers do not participate in learning and educating themselves about the disease or illness trajectory. Rather, the Carrier caregiver looks to the healthcare team to provide access to information on the disease, seeks information limited to disease treatment and ongoing care, and conveys comprehensive understanding of the healthcare system. However, given the LOW/WARM conversation pattern, they are highly avoidant of prognosis information as a way of coping with the illness (Lee et al., 2018). Information seeking and suppression is a common coping mechanism for the Carrier caregiver who limits question asking to topics pertaining to physical care for the care recipient, how to make them comfortable, and how to make caregiving more efficient and better. Active information-seeking is tied to the quality of caregiving.

In the following example, a caregiver describes her uncertainty about caring for her sister following a double mastectomy:

I had to be the one to change all the draining tube(s). And I wasn't for sure if I was doing it right, because I never went to a class. I was just thrown into this. It was like I never knew anything about cancer. I would go on the Internet and just make sure I was doing the draining tubes right. I looked for what type of food that would help her, such as you know, the green vegetables, such as broccoli. What to give her to help her iron, because she had a poor iron deficiency. And she had to have blood transfusions twice under my care. So, she moved in with me. That's where the Internet came in for me, to see if, to find the dos and the don'ts. You know, what is it, that she should be eating, should she be exercising? If she had problems with anything, I would go in there and look to see, should I call the doctor now? Should I take her to the hospital now? Things like that that I was faced with.

Realizing that she had not been trained for providing this type of care at home and that she had limited knowledge about cancer, this caregiver turned to the Internet for information. However, she sought only information about draining the tubes, nutrition, and exercise, all focused specific caregiving tasks and promoting healthy well-being. Her information needs did not involve learning more about the disease and prognosis, and she describes her communication challenges pertaining to care. This restricted approach to information, and limited use of healthcare team members for learning more, creates communication challenges for the Carrier caregiver.

SELF-CARE AND THE CARRIER

Following the family's traditional expectations for caregiving, the Carrier caregiver accepts caregiving responsibilities without question and with little regard for their own self-care needs (Guo et al., 2019). With the primary focus on the needs of the care recipient, the Carrier caregiver becomes disconnected from their own self-care needs. Daniel describes this:

There was really no time to react in the moment [diagnosis], I was in shock and extremely worried about how my grandma would take the news. But, later on when I was alone it really did hit hard on my heart. I had no time to really process it because I had to take care of my grandma, I'm still kind of processing the whole thing, sometimes it feels like I'm in some sort of very unrealistic dream.

There is little time or space for the Carrier caregiver to contemplate anything other than their caregiving role:

I have to do a lot of the caregiving myself; my mother and aunt help out as well but for the most part my family expects me to be there for my grandma. I take her to doctor's appointments, buy her medication, and spend any free time I have taking care of her; most of my cousins or aunts and uncles rarely stop by.

There is no talk about what is expected within the family, and no one is acting except the caregiver. The invisibility of their labors is common for the Carrier caregiver due to HIGH/COLD conformity patterns where obligation is prioritized. Carrier caregivers underscore their strength and ability to handle caregiving, repeatedly pointing out that they are capable of handling the patient's psychological stress. Explanations for the patient's feelings (e.g., anger, frustration, sadness) and empathy for the patient's illness are frequent topics for the Carrier caregiver and used to prioritize quality patient care over caregiver self-care.

Caregiving remains a prominently task-driven activity for the Carrier who disguises caregiving within the family system without talking about it directly. While it is okay for the care recipient to thank the caregiver for quality care and duty to family, it is not okay to talk about the disease itself, the future, or caregiving stress. To talk about it is a violation of privacy boundaries for the Carrier's family:

Whenever I see my family they might bring it up [illness] for a couple of minutes, but I think everybody is just too sad or uncomfortable to talk about it. Most of them want to just ignore it. . . . We do not talk about things like [if treatment doesn't work] ever. I think about it a lot but there is never anybody in my family that wants to listen. They call me a jerk or insensitive for even bringing it up but I think I am just being realistic, honestly.

Daniel recognizes that talk about his grandma's illness is taboo within his family. The family establishes allowable topics that include a focus on health, cure, and getting better and dismisses talk about treatment, caregiving, and preparation for future decisions. These conversations are too difficult for the Carrier's family system. Thus, the disease can be discussed but in a limited way that prioritizes family functioning.

As a result, Carrier caregivers report the lowest health literacy in the area of self-care (Wittenberg et al., 2017). Among some cultures, seeking assistance would not be considered appropriate as cultural beliefs influence whether or not caregiver self-care is culturally appropriate. A strong cultural justification for caregiving limits the Carrier's self-care behaviors, self-care resource use, and communication about self-care. Carrier caregivers would feel guilty if they had personal autonomy about their day or time away from caregiving. The Carrier caregiver does not directly communicate personal needs to other family members nor seek formal support. Carrier caregivers with high family obligation may have an avoidant attachment style as caregiving is accepted as legitimate work (Lee et al., 2018). Caregiving is fulfilling to the Carrier caregiver, despite high avoidance within the family.

SUMMARY

For the Carrier caregiver, caregiving is an opportunity to fulfill family duty and demonstrate family commitment through sacrifice and hard work. A HIGH/ COLD conformity pattern reveals an obligation to care for other family members, an implicit understanding that illness requires immediate family mobilization, and a belief that gatekeeping is necessary to sustain and preserve family functioning. The LOW/WARM conversation pattern exposes unclear rules for talking about illness. There is inconsistency in topics discussed, ideas are disjointed, and specific circumstances when talk about illness is considered permissible. Self-restraint among family members inhibits open sharing, and nondisclosure is considered honoring family. As *protector of the care* recipient, the Carrier caregiver is task-driven and focuses on keeping the illness a private family experience. Box 6.1 summarizes the Carrier caregiver across the topics explored in this chapter.

CODA

Carrier caregivers are often solo caregivers who shoulder the bulk of all caregiving responsibilities. As solo caregiving is also common among spouses caring for individuals with dementia, it is likely that many of these caregivers are Carrier caregivers (Ornstein et al., 2019). Challenges for caregivers of patients with chronic illness are exacerbated when the chronic illness is dementia. Approximately 15 million U.S. family caregivers provide unpaid support for loved ones with dementia, yet little has been done to integrate caregiver support into the routine care of these patients (Slaboda et al., 2018). Caregivers of individuals with dementia also mistrust the healthcare system. Despite increases in advance care planning, only 40% of individuals with dementia undertake advance care planning (Sellars

Box 6.1

Family Communication Pattern
- Conformity—High, Cold
- Conversation—Low, Warm
- Caregiver surmises other family members' needs during caregiving

Behaviors in the Illness Process
- Presents to others as *protector of the care recipient*
- Highlights personal strength to handle caregiving tasks

Family Expectations for Caregiving
- Cultural, social obligation to parents and elders
- Feelings of indebtedness to care recipient

Family Roles
- Caregiving is solitary role
- Tendency to avoid stressful discussions about illness with all
- Serve as sounding board for care recipient

Family Decision-Making
- Accommodate care recipient with focus on physical needs and medication regimens
- Family decision-making does not occur without healthcare provider involvement

Family Uncertainty
- Worry about caregiving performance

Palliative Care Communication and Health Literacy Considerations
- Responsive to directions and high achieving
- Limits information-seeking to caregiving tasks, not illness information
- Healthcare team is primary source of information
- Does not share information with care recipient
- Palliative care approach should focus on caregiver relationship with care recipient

Self-Care
- Does not talk about caregiving role with family members
- Information seeking and suppression are common coping mechanisms
- Feels guilty receiving support from others
- Lowest self-care and highest uncertainty

et al., 2019), and they often receive suboptimal end-of-life care and are more likely to receive overly aggressive treatment.

REFERENCES

Aloweni, F., Doshi, K., Fook-Chong, S., Malhotra, R., & Ostbye, T. (2019). The types of caregiving reactions experienced by the older spouse caregivers. *Journal of Clinical Nursing, 28*(23-24), 4538–4548. https://doi.org/10.1111/jocn.15044

Benson, J. J., Parker Oliver, D., Demiris, G., & Washington, K. (2019). Accounts of family conflict in home hospice care: The central role of autonomy for informal caregiver resilience. *Journal of Family Nursing, 25*(2), 190–218. https://doi.org/10.1177/1074840719828091

Campesino, M., Saenz, D. S., Choi, M., & Krouse, R. S. (2012). Perceived discrimination and ethnic identity among breast cancer survivors. *Oncology Nursing Forum, 39*(2), E91–E100. https://doi.org/10.1188/12.ONF.E91-E100

Coelho, A., de Brito, M., Teixeira, P., Frade, P., Barros, L., & Barbosa, A. (2019). Family caregivers' anticipatory grief: A conceptual framework for understanding its multiple challenges. *Qualitative Health Research, 30*(5), 693–703. https://doi.org/10.1177/1049732319873330

Costas-Muniz, R., Sen, R., Leng, J., Aragones, A., Ramirez, J., & Gany, F. (2013). Cancer stage knowledge and desire for information: Mismatch in Latino cancer patients? *Journal of Cancer Education, 28*(3), 458–465. https://doi.org/10.1007/s13187-013-0487-8

Dark-Freudeman, A., Greskovich, L., & Terry, C. (2016). The relationship between attachment style, depressive symptoms, and social support: A survey of caregivers. *Educational Gerontology, 42*(2), 89–99.

Eliassen, A. H. (2016). Power relations and health care communication in older adulthood: Educating recipients and providers. *Gerontologist, 56*(6), 990–996. https://doi.org/10.1093/geront/gnv095

Evans, B. C., Coon, D. W., Belyea, M. J., & Ume, E. (2017). Collective care: Multiple caregivers and multiple care recipients in Mexican American families. *Journal of Transcultural Nursing, 28*(4), 398–407. https://doi.org/10.1177/1043659616657878

Goldsmith, J., Wittenberg, E., Platt, C., Iannarino, N., & Reno, J. (2015). Family caregiver communication: Advancing a typology. *Psycho-Oncology, 25*(4), 463–470. https://doi.org/10.1002/pon.3862

Guo, M., Kim, S. H., & Dong, X. (2019). Sense of filial obligation and caregiving burdens among Chinese immigrants in the United States. *Journal of the American Geriatric Society, 6*, S564–S570.

Heyzer, L., Alli, N. B., Chew, A. P., Chan, M., & Lim, W. S. (2019). Worry about performance: Unravelling the relationship between "doing more" and "doing better." *Journal of Nutrition, Health, and Aging, 23*(9), 843–848.

Laidsaar-Powell, R., Butow, P., Charles, C., Gafni, A., Entwistle, V., Epstein, R., & Juraskova, I. (2017). The TRIO framework: Conceptual insights into family caregiver involvement and influence throughout cancer treatment decision-making. *Patient and Education Counseling, 100*(11), 2035–2046. https://doi.org/10.1016/j.pec.2017.05.014

Lee, J., Sohn, B. K., Lee, H., Seong, S. J., Park, S., & Lee, J. Y. (2018). Attachment style and filial obligation in the burden of caregivers of dementia patients. *Archives of Gerontology & Geriatrics, 75*, 104–111. https://doi.org/10.1016/j.archger.2017.12.002

Lim, W. S., Cheah, W. K., Ali, N., Han, H. C., Anthony, P. V., Chan, M., & Chong, M. S. (2014). Worry about performance: A unique dimension of caregiver burden. *International Psychogeriatrics, 26*(4), 677–686.

Liu, J., & Bern-Klug, M. (2016). "I should be doing more for my parent:" Chinese adult children's worry about performance in providing care for their oldest-old parents. *International Psychogeriatrics, 28*(2), 303–315.

Mead, E. L., Doorenbos, A. Z., Javid, S. H., Haozous, E. A., Alvord, L. A., Flum, D. R., & Morris, A. M. (2013). Shared decision-making for cancer care among racial and ethnic minorities: A systematic review. *American Journal of Public Health, 103*(12), e15–e29. https://doi.org/10.2105/AJPH.2013.301631

Ornstein, K. A., Wolff, J. L., Bollens-Lund, E., Rahman, O. K., & Kelley, A. S. (2019). Spousal caregivers are caregiving alone in the last years of life. *Health Affairs (Millwood), 38*(6), 964–972. https://doi.org/10.1377/hlthaff.2019.00087

Paulson, D., & Bassett, R. (2016). Prepared to care: Adult attachment and filial obligation. *Aging & Mental Health, 20*(11), 1221–1228. https://doi.org/10.1080/13607863.2015.1072800

Pharr, J., Francis, C. D., Terry, C., & Clark, M. C. (2014). Culture, caregiving, and health: Exploring the influence of culture on family caregiver experiences. *ISRN Public Health, 2014*(Article ID 689826). https://doi.org/http://dx.doi.org/10.1155/2014/689826

Roberto, K. A., McCann, B. R., Blieszner, R., & Savla, J. (2019). A long and winding road: Dementia caregiving with grit and grace. *Innovation in Aging, 3*(3), igz021. https://doi.org/10.1093/geroni/igz021

Roeland, E., Cain, J., Onderdonk, C., Kerr, K., Mitchell, W., & Thornberry, K. (2014). When open-ended questions don't work: The role of palliative paternalism in difficult medical decisions. *Journal of Palliative Medicine, 17*(4), 415–420. https://doi.org/10.1089/jpm.2013.0408

Sellars, M., Chung, O., Nolte, L., Tong, A., Pond, D., Fetherstonhaugh, D., . . . Detering, K. M. (2019). Perspectives of people with dementia and carers on advance care planning and end-of-life care: A systematic review and thematic synthesis of qualitative studies. *Palliative Medicine, 33*(3), 274–290. https://doi.org/10.1177/0269216318809571

Slaboda, J., Fail, R., Norman, G. J., & Meier, D. E. (2018, January 11). A study of family caregiver burden and the imperative of practice change to address family caregivers' unmet needs. *Health Affairs Blog.* https://www.healthaffairs.org/do/10.1377/hblog20180105.914873/full/

Wiebe, W. T., Zhang, Y. B., & Liu, N. (2018). Intergenerational conflict management styles: Exploring the indirect effects of sex through filial obligation. *China Media Research, 14*(3), 44–56.

Wittenberg, E., Goldsmith, J. V., & Kerr, A. M. (2019). Variation in health literacy among family caregiver communication types. *Psycho-Oncology, 28*(11), 2181–2187. https://doi.org/10.1002/pon.5204

Wittenberg, E., Kravits, K., Goldsmith, J., Ferrell, B., & Fujinami, R. (2017). Validation of a model of family caregiver communication types and related caregiver outcomes. *Palliative & Supportive Care*, *15*(1), 3–11. https://doi.org/10.1017/ S1478951516000109

Wittenberg-Lyles, E., Goldsmith, J., Demiris, G., Oliver, D. P., & Stone, J. (2012). The impact of family communication patterns on hospice family caregivers: A new typology. *Journal of Hospice & Palliative Nursing*, *14*(1), 25–33. https://doi.org/ 10.1097/NJH.0b013e318233114b

Zhang, X., Clarke, C. L., & Rhynas, S. J. (2019). What is the meaning of filial piety for people with dementia and their family caregivers in China under the current so-cial traditions? An interpretive phenomenological analysis. *Dementia*, *18*(7–8), 2620–2634.

Spotlight

Desire for Best Possible Care

A pressing issue for caregivers is finding the balance between pushing their loved ones to do what they consider best for their health and respecting how their care recipient's desire to live after being diagnosed with serious illness. Lucy expressed guilt about nagging her sedentary husband to get more exercise in an attempt to forestall his dementia: "He could be thwarting his disease by working out." Admittedly active all the time, she has little patience with Chuck's sitting and his refusal to exercise at the pace and intensity that she sees as a possible antidote to the progression of his illness. And she is the one who has meticulously researched his disease and has discovered that physical activity may indeed be helpful.

Yet her nagging is hurtful to both of them, Lucy realizes, and she is unforgiving of her aggressive "meanness," which he has let her know he resents. "I can't blow up at somebody who's developing dementia," she laments. She is striving to find that balance between giving him the benefit of her extensive research into his disease while also being a loving, patient partner who can understand that he deserves to be responsible for his own decisions about how to live his life. What she believes about her caregiving role collides with her ideals about being a good wife. "How far do you push someone to take care of themselves?" is a question Lucy must have asked prior to Chuck's diagnosis; his disease has greatly enhanced its stakes.

Carolina, who has cared for Waldo for many months as he has progressed to hospice care, also wishes to be her husband's best possible caregiver. Because Waldo is now bedbound, Carolina's pride in caring for him is confined to providing him with elemental needs: "The most wonderful thing I can do for Waldo is to make sure that he's comfortable and he's clean and dry and he's safe at home with us." She works hard at caregiving to ascertain that "when Waldo is gone, I can look at it and know I did my best. I did everything I could for him. That means a lot to me." Her goals are realistic and of the moment; while the roles of caregiver and spouse may have been in conflict occasionally in the initial phases of Waldo's disease, there is now certainty that she is caring for him in the best ways possible.

Carolina has also found comfort in framing her caregiving as an opportunity for teaching others about how to care for a loved one at home. As a former nurse, Carolina is a natural instructor; she also trained several professional caregiving agency caregivers how to care for her husband at their home when these caregivers lacked the specific skills needed. She believes strongly in the goodness of caring for sick and dying family members in the comfort of their own homes:

> I feel like in a sense I'm teaching: I put it on Facebook: what we're doing and why we're doing it and what this journey is because I feel like this is how life is. . . . We're doing a great disservice to our family members if we have the resources and wherewithal to care for them when they're in hospice in their final days.

Carolina offers to give her friends any help they might need with their own caregiving tasks and the resources to help them because she feels the effort is so worthwhile. "I just think that if we as humans understand that death is part of life and it's expected, and we're all dying of the same disease, the lack of immortality—that's a 'Waldoism'—with hospice care we're doing 'now care' and 'now care' includes joy." Carolina meets regularly with friends who are experiencing caregiving challenges and has heard from so many who are struggling with caregiving issues similar to the ones she has faced. She gives them advice for the problems they may face as their loved ones' disease advances and they approach death: She calls this "anticipatory guidance" and includes such pragmatic suggestions as the kind of adult diapers their care receivers may need. Facebook has served her well in this quest as she adamantly believes in "getting the story out there" to help the next person. Carolina is also eager to help hospice workers know the right equipment to use that helps patients find comfort in their dying; for example, a neck pillow and a memory foam layer on a mattress to prevent bedsores—"little tricks that I feel I can share with someone to make their life easier." Still, she acknowledges that caregiving is an isolating, exhausting, often tedious task—and one that interferes with personal freedoms that are sorely missed in the course of nonstop caring for another.

Being the best possible caregiver to a loved one is a mission that guides many caregivers' lives. Most struggle, however, to find that balance that preserves the self while also catering to the other—and of continuing to manifest love while also witnessing the physical and mental decline of the beloved. The uncertainty of disease trajectories and concomitant stress and anxiety for both parties exacerbate the caregiving challenge. Yet family caregivers are quick to assert that "you have to treasure all the times you have together" and "you have to create joy for the rest of the life you have together."

7

The Partner Caregiver

We openly talk about it [cancer] even when she's around, and we want to make sure, you know, we have solutions. We know that she's on chemotherapy, and we also find holistic ways to try to make her feel better and, you know, her mind as well, to stay positive. I think that describes us really well. And I want to say "us" because I feel like I'm not the only caregiver. We're all, we're all just partners, and we're all a team going through.

—Lou, best friend of Val, cancer patient

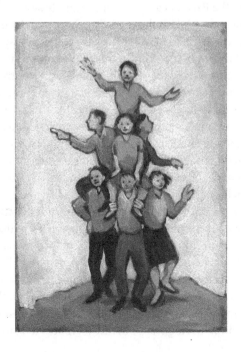

In this chapter's opening illustration by Aust, the individuals on the bottom of the pyramid are not braced for the heaviness of their tasks; instead, they are willing partners who invite others onto their shoulders for the journey. For the Partner caregiver, individuals collectively create a "pyramid of support" without each person knowing, asking, requiring, or even realizing it. The simplicity of the family structure does not reveal tension or stress but rather a coming together that enables a wide variety of perspectives to be shared and the lack of an intense focus on direction. Each person is looking through their own lens, in their own direction, and is not worried about what the others are doing. The Partner caregiver, positioned at the top, does not feel the grip of family beneath or the stress from others who bear her weight. This foundation affords the Partner caregiver the ability to focus on the care recipient and their own emotions about loss and caregiving and to dive deep into the difficult conversations about overwhelming change, illness, and adjustment. In this chapter, the Partner caregiver is described within a family system where the chronic illness experience gives family members an opportunity to learn to adapt the family system, cooperate with each other, engage in emotions about caregiving, act together as a family, balance roles, and encourage each other (Anderson & White, 2018).

FAMILY COMMUNICATION PATTERNS OF THE PARTNER CAREGIVER

LOW/WARM conformity and HIGH/WARM conversation communication patterns give rise to the Partner caregiver whose family system shares in open and frequent communication while at the same time values family member independence (Wittenberg, Kravits, et al., 2017). The care recipient–caregiver relationship is the embodiment of family harmony in this LOW conformity pattern, and each family member is allowed to experience the illness differently and in their own way. Typical partner caregiver–care recipient relationships include adult children caring for a parent or spousal caregivers where there has been a long-standing pattern of open communication between the two individuals. HIGH/WARM conversation patterns create a comfortable communication climate for family members to explicitly name and talk about illness, directly acknowledging that illness is the cause of change within the family, and enable conversations about a variety of topics including death and dying, spirituality, and quality of life.

Family members do not feel obligated to spend time together; rather, family time emerges from conversation among family members, which reflects a LOW/WARM conformity pattern. In a LOW/WARM conformity pattern, there are no family rules for what is expected during a family member's illness. While family members share a unified concern for the care recipient, they do not feel obligated to act in the same way by mobilizing physically. Instead, family members come together with no family leader or expectations for family presence. Family mobilization results from the willingness of family members to come together anyway they want, either physically, by phone, sending text messages, or via videoconference. All of these are acceptable formats because there is diversity in attitudes and beliefs among family members about how they should mobilize. WARM conformity patterns are also characterized by a variety of support provided. Because independence is valued, family members only expect each other to give what they are able in terms of support, be it financial, emotional, or physical support. Partner caregivers appreciate and welcome family involvement, recognizing that support will be composed of many miscellaneous parts. With a value on autonomy, family members' other commitments are acknowledged as just as important as family need, regardless of whether or not these commitments are work, their own family, or social/personal commitments. Alone time is also honored, and personal space is valued.

A patchwork of ideas is shared between family members about the care recipient's illness and needs, and there is diversity in the subjects covered, representing a HIGH/WARM conversation pattern. This pattern supports spontaneous open conversation among family members about the illness and various kinds of ideas are shared and considered. Each family member has license to share their ideas and concerns freely, including Partner caregivers who can vocalize their fears and concerns and can share the changes that occur throughout the illness. Frequent and spontaneous conversation occurs among family members, allowing the family to share knowledge and resources and to plan ahead for care needs. This characteristic of an open system shows potential to discuss a variety of topics such as advance care planning, which increases connections. This does not mean that Partner caregivers never experience family conflict, only that conflict is discussed openly. A HIGH/WARM conversation pattern prioritizes shared decision-making among family members and the realization that compromise is necessary. In chronic illness, compromise is influenced by the values and beliefs of the care recipient, which are often shared by the care recipient or Partner caregiver as a result of open communication patterns.

PARTNER BEHAVIORS IN THE ILLNESS PROCESS

In contrast with the Carrier and Manager caregiver types, the onset of disease generates increased family communication for the Partner caregiver rather than increased family member presence. Mobilization of the family occurs in a variety of formats, determined by the individual family member as to what is the best way and time for them to come together with family and the care recipient. An unexpected diagnosis that comes on quickly (acute) may prompt more immediate attention and frequent communication among family members, but family members do not necessarily feel compelled to show up in person because of an acute situation. Open and frequent communication is the backbone of this family system, so mobilization occurs through family text messaging, private Facebook groups, other social media outlets, and group phone calls. When the onset of disease is more gradual and occurs over time, family members also refer to open communication patterns to discuss and compare notes about what has been observed with the care recipient. The Partner caregiver presents to others as the *supporter of the experiences of the care recipient,* providing confirmation of the physical and emotional changes taking place. Given the emphasis on open communication, initiating topics about the health of the care recipient is viewed as natural and allowable and as a way of conveying family support. But, again, this does not immediately trigger family mobilization; rather, it fortifies family commitment through conversation. Conversations then lead to family adaptation as roles and responsibilities among family members emerge to support care.

While Carrier caregivers entrench themselves in high-intensity caregiving regardless of the illness trajectory, the Partner caregiver experiences a range of high- and low-intensity caregiving as determined by the course of disease. The reciprocal experience between care recipient and Partner caregiver creates an ebb and flow to caregiving with increased family support presence when needed and less family presence when not needed. In a constant disease course, such as cancer, which can include periods of stabilization and survivorship, there are periods of recovery for the Partner caregiver as the care recipient takes the lead in living. Similarly, in relapsing or episodic disease courses such as type 2 diabetes or multiple sclerosis, periods of stabilization allow the caregiver to back off from caregiving responsibilities. In more progressive disease courses such as Alzheimer's disease, the Partner caregiver is able to utilize the support of family members when they need it. Family members are "on call" and easily and readily accept a role in supporting the Partner caregiver's respite needs. Family adaptation to chronic illness is more readily put into place for Partner caregivers; the range in caregiving intensity results from (a) the family's ability to honor the care recipient's decisions for care and ways of living even when they disagree and (b) the family's ability to combine characteristics among family members, which allows family members to be on standby until needed.

While Manager and Carrier caregivers may be more inclined to maintain hope by dispelling, avoiding, or ignoring information about care, the Partner caregiver is committed to understanding and discussing the outcome of the disease by asking about end-of-life care and end-of-disease trajectory. This does not mean that these conversations are not difficult, just that Partner caregivers are more likely to be willing to discuss the "big picture" of the chronic illness. They are not overzealous in their information seeking yet may initiate a discussion about end-of-life care or prognosis even when healthcare providers are uncomfortable. Prognostic uncertainty is less impactful for the Partner caregiver because the family's focus is on the care recipient's wishes and quality of life. Understanding the disease is vital to engaging in advanced care planning and helping the care recipient with decision-making. The Partner caregiver shares all information received about the illness with the care recipient. There is little need to protect others from this information as the Partner caregiver and family feel empowered knowing the "truth" of the diagnosis, the "truth" of the prognosis, and the "truth" of what the illness journey will look like toward the end. This is tricky in chronic illness where there is no clear trajectory for the disease.

Within the family system, there can be another family member who gathers the information and shares it with the Partner caregiver. Unlike other caregiver types who may be the sole recipient of communication and information from healthcare providers, the Partner caregiver may actually get information second-hand from another family member who has engaged healthcare staff as the family spokesperson. In this way, the Partner caregiver may receive illness information from a close and trusted family member. Boundaries are protected by sharing information with each other in ways that have previously been proven successful and acceptable for sharing family communication. Not all family members are able to accept information in the same way, and many engage in different information-seeking strategies and trust different sources of information. Conflict can exist but open communication keeps family members focused on the care recipient's needs and wishes and the need to share all with the family.

As the care recipient's physical and cognitive functioning slip away, the family utilizes the assorted contributions of many family members to constantly adjust. For the Partner caregiver's family system, concerns for the care recipient and the caregiver are equally discussed in the family's approach and adaptation to chronic illness. Coping and stress are shared openly and respectfully, even with the care recipient. Uniquely, the Partner caregiver is deeply affected by the degree to which the care recipient becomes incapacitated. Unlike Carrier caregivers who struggle with family functioning and fulfilling their family role as well as the care recipient's family duties, the Partner caregiver begins to experience the loss of the care recipient who has provided emotional support. The need for emotional support is exacerbated by this loss over the duration of the illness.

FAMILY EXPECTATIONS FOR CAREGIVING

The Partner caregiver's family system values family member independence and autonomy, so when a family member is diagnosed with a chronic illness, there is no pressure for any one individual in the family to step into the caregiving role and no pressure for how this caregiver should perform caregiving responsibilities. HIGH/WARM conversation patterns, which are the predominant communication pattern for Partner caregivers, shape the family's view of the health situation as a shared challenge. Chronic illness is not considered a "personal experience" that impacts the care recipient; it is viewed as a shared experience that impacts the person who is ill and the family member whom they are closest to. This close, intimate relationship between care recipient and family member segues into the Partner caregiving role.

Deiondre

It became just gradually that I was taking on more and more. In 2016 he was hospitalized for 16 days and after that he was in rehab for 40 days and at that point that's when I began to take on full responsibility for his care. . . . He has severe [chronic obstructive pulmonary disease]. At this stage he has to be on oxygen 24/7. He has to take, do his nebulizer treatment about every four hours when he's awake. He has an inhaler, a rescue inhaler that he uses when he feels extreme shortness of breath that, especially after excursions. So anytime he finds himself struggling he can use that inhaler.

Deiondre cares for her husband of 56 years and explains how she slowly found herself in the caregiving role. For the Partner caregiver, the mutual engagement of managing chronic illness includes assuming responsibility for the patient, participating in decision-making processes, being informed, and learning ways to provide care (Reigada et al., 2015). While there may be a cultural background that sets cultural expectations (e.g., "family values" to help one another or "being raised to help one another") particularly for spousal and adult children caregivers, expectations for caregiving for the Partner caregiver are not culturally driven but are more about relational closeness.

Relationship type (e.g., spouse, child) and quality impact caregiving roles and expectations for families with HIGH conversation and LOW conformity (Reblin et al., 2019). Relationship quality has been characterized by warmth, closeness, and support or hostility, conflict, and distance (Bouchard et al., 2019) and impacts whether or not caregivers see their role as unwanted and confining and whether or not they feel they can manage the responsibility (Bangerter et al., 2019). When the caregiver and patient have high relationship quality, the caregiver is more likely to feel they can manage the responsibility and desire the caregiving role. The distinctive feature of HIGH/WARM patterns in the family system sustains high relational quality between Partner caregiver and care recipient. Partner caregivers naturally assume the caregiving role because of their close connection with the care recipient.

Relationship quality can be highly influenced by cultural expectations for family and family member relationships, as seen in the examples in Box 7.1.

Where cultural expectations within the family of origin drive the caregiving role for the Carrier caregiver, the Partner caregiver does not experience pressure or expectations from within the family system. However, some Partner caregivers like Esme, experience pressure coming from outside the family origin:

I remember from when my mother was first diagnosed. It was a constant communication with our family outside of the [United States] because our family here is very limited. . . . So, it was just a lot of phone calls and a lot of my aunts and my uncles reminding me that I'm the only family she has here. So, it is my responsibility to take care of her and since I am the oldest, the oldest from my siblings. . . . I have a responsibility to take care of my mother.

Esme's mother was diagnosed with breast cancer and, over the last two years, has had surgery, chemotherapy, and now radiation. She describes how it was hard to hear this from "the people who aren't here to help out":

Box 7.1

PARTNER DESCRIPTIONS OF THE RELATIONSHIP WITH THE CARE RECIPIENT
(2019 DATA COLLECTIONS)

- *I talk to him like an old friend. We don't always see eye-to-eye on things but he knows that I just want the best for him.* (Cancer patient, son caregiver)
- *I was raised in a loving home although absent from my father she was the main parent and that's how the relationship built and is so strong.* (Stroke patient, daughter caregiver)
- *He knows that I'm here, he relies on me, but I wouldn't put it terms of he expects me to do it. Yes and no, it's kind of strange to you know he knows that I'm here for him I'll put it that way, he knows that.* (COPD patient, spouse caregiver)
- *He's my dad so I feel pretty close to him. I come from a very large Italian family so family it's kind of the center of our culture. It's common for siblings to take care of their parents as they get older. . . . If he's around I want to make sure that I'm not going to reveal stuff that is going to embarrass him or that he's going to feel self-conscious about. When I have time alone with him I can be a little bit more candid.* (Dementia patient, son caregiver)

It made me feel a bit resentful. Because it is hard to just hear all these comments about how it's my responsibility to take care of my mother. Which I honestly you know, I take the responsibility and I'm willing to, I have been willing to help my mother. But it also made me feel and question where the support from my family on the outside was coming from, just having them tell me that I have to take care of my mom was a lot to take in, and I felt I was alone in this situation. I felt I needed more people to reach out and come here and help me caregive for my mother.

Expectations for caregiving from family members do not motivate the Partner caregiver (as they do the Carrier caregiver) and in this case Esme's resentment grows deep. The willingness for caregiving comes from the closeness with the care recipient and differentiates the Partner from the Carrier caregiver whose motivation stems primarily from family obligation.

The relationship quality between the caregiver and care recipient largely influences whether a family member is a Partner caregiver. Emotional support, closeness, and a joint adaptable response based on shared relationship history are key indicators of a high quality relationship (Conway et al., 2018). Between care recipient and Partner caregiver, there is an expectation that illness information will be openly shared and discussed as part of caregiving efforts, as examples in Box 7.2 illustrate. Close emotional bonds, often explained by attachment theory, support a family communication climate where illness conversations occur openly.

Box 7.2

Partner Descriptions of Shared Knowledge With Care Recipient (2019 Data Collections)

- *I don't learn anything new that she, that we don't share together. I always go with her for all of her treatments, all of her doctor visits. So I'm not learning anything that she doesn't already know. . . . Although, I would default to her in, in maybe in some instances, but we talk it through to make sure that that's the best decision.* (Cancer patient, spouse caregiver)
- *We walk side by side, I can't . . . I don't force him into anything. I suggest things. If he wants to pooh-pooh it, he pooh-poohs it. If he wants to go with it, he goes with it. But we don't, you know, we're not like that . . . we talk about everything.* (Cancer patient, spouse caregiver)
- *We love each other and so everything we do is the result of our love for one another he often expresses regret that he can't do what he used to do and I do my best to reassure him that what he does is a blessing anyway and you know we are Christians and that always fits into the picture of how we behave with one another.* (COPD patient, spouse caregiver)

FAMILY ROLES

In the Partner caregiver family system, caregiving is considered a team effort where every member has a role and ability to contribute. New family routines and communicating with one another are all aspects of family functioning that are present for the Partner caregiver (Zhang, 2018), as described in Box 7.3.

Role stability, connectivity, and family resources are all positively affected by the family's open communication process (Kim et al., 2018). The Partner caregiver does not organize, schedule, or plan for family communication. It just happens. The family moves into action, sometimes rallying behind the Partner caregiver who works independently but with family support and sometimes as a larger unit with multiple family members working together to accomplish caregiving tasks. Distance between family members is easily overcome by the Partner caregiver who shares resources available through the healthcare system with others (Wittenberg, Buller, et al., 2017).

The family's role in chronic illness management includes open conversations about disease in day-to-day family living. Family communication includes "turning to" the reality of the disease by engaging in conversations about roles within the family system (Colquhoun et al., 2019). Chronic illness becomes part of family conversation, as illustrated in Miguel's recollection of the day he learned about his mother's diagnosis:

It was one day after work. . . . I just got home. It was like any other day. She just pulled me aside for a quick minute and she just told me the news: 'Oh

Box 7.3

PARTNER DESCRIPTIONS OF FAMILY ADAPTATION TO CHRONIC ILLNESS (2019 DATA COLLECTIONS)

- *There are six of us that are involved in doing this. Two that take care of her during the day and the other four, we take care of her in the evening, we all go off and on in the evening and on the weekends and that way the other two, they have the weekends off. We talk and we share information frequently. My sister who usually takes her to the doctors, she contacts us and lets us know if there is any kind of a change. (Alzheimer's patient, daughter caregiver)*
- *We're all pretty involved, like me, and her dad, and her family, and our close friends. We all take turns, and we all—I mean, although I always want to be there, I know that we all have lives, and we all have to, you know, have—go to our jobs, and do different things on the weekends, and get to what we have to get done, and have a little time for ourselves as well and she [care recipient] knows as well. She's always asking how we're doing, and we try not to always just talk about the cancer. And we're all very helpful with each other as, as far as, like, time and what we do for her. And I think it's—so far it's been very good, the way we all communicate. (Cancer patient, best friend caregiver)*
- *We get together as a family and make the decision (regarding treatment). We don't just leave it to one person. We talk about it." (Alzheimer's patient, sister caregiver)*
- *When I am tired I tell them to take over for me for a while. Sometimes I need a break because it is usually the same routine every day. (Patient with Type 2 diabetes, niece caregiver)*

hey, I just came back from the doctor's and they diagnosed me with type 2 diabetes.' It was a little overwhelming at first. . . . There's been a history of diabetes [in the family]. . . . It's just brought us closer because it's something that there's a high chance that we will develop. There's always concern for it. . . . My grandma and my mom they always tell me watch out, watch out what you eat, try to avoid certain [foods] because it's obviously high risk in our family.

The nonchalant nature of his mother's diagnosis, shared casually the same day she received it, became a family topic. Unplanned, ordinary communication about disease between family members is characteristic of the Partner family system. When a prolonged disease trajectory is anticipated and there are genetic implications, the disease is recognized as a family disease and talk about the disease is normalized within the family.

An important family role of the Partner caregiver is to support the care recipient by helping to manage the disease. The Manager and Carrier caregiver commonly approach the caregiving role by directly overseeing the care recipient's self-management responsibilities such as medication regimens. In contrast, the Partner caregiver's goal is to help remind the patient about the day-to-day requirements of chronic illness management. Miguel explains his goal for supporting his mother as she manages type 2 diabetes:

> I wanna be there for her . . . so she can be herself . . . to not let this illness get the best of her. Sometimes she forgets and so I have to remind her, but most of the times she's good on her own. She looks things up or she asks at the doctor's or something. But for the most part she basically does it on her own but she forgets sometimes.

The Partner caregiver considers the caregiving role as complementary to the care recipient rather than as the person responsible for all aspects of care.

Partner caregivers attend to and are mindful of the emotional support needed in chronic care management. They work to minimize or manage patient suffering by providing emotional support, keeping the patient's hope up, carrying out the patient's wishes, and communicating empathy and understanding (Reigada et al., 2015). A spousal caregiver who assists her husband with managing his positive HIV status explains how she does this:

> If you miss a dose, sometime he'll get real nervous, "Oh, I have anxiety attack. I done miss this and missed that." I said, well, just take an extra one, you know, so I just told him you'll be all right. One dose ain't going to hurt you. . . . I let him know that I'm here . . . keep him motivated . . . being there for him. . . . My biggest struggle, when they get depressed and I had to motivate him all back over again. Look, you're gone too far.

The Partner caregiver and care recipient enjoy a close, intimate relationship, which allows the caregiver to provide direct patient support through encouragement and compassion. Partner caregivers who willingly volunteer to serve as caregiver because of a deep emotional connection with the care recipient are more likely to have the psychological or cognitive flexibility to respond more effectively to situational demands (Jen et al., 2019). Providing emotional support is naturally part of the caregiving role and a unique factor in the Partner caregiver's adjustment to the demands of the illness and social support (Hou et al., 2018).

FAMILY DECISION-MAKING

Just as family roles are adopted by each family member in an effort to contribute to caregiving and support Partner caregiving efforts, the family system also embraces a collective family approach to decision-making. Although LOW/WARM conformity patterns are present, family values set expectations that the family will make decisions together, revealing a WARM conformity pattern that supports family harmony. Integrated into this shared approach is a general sense of trusting physicians to guide them in the decision-making process. Ultimately, however, it is the Partner caregiver's family system that debriefs together to make sure that each family member agrees and feels comfortable with the decision. Central to this process is the role of family in discussing information given by healthcare providers with the care recipient (Wittenberg-Lyles, Goldsmith, Demiris et al., 2012), demonstrating the family emphasis on open communication patterns. Box 7.4 illustrates examples of the Partner caregiver's unified family approach to decision-making.

Emphasizing family harmony through collective efforts involves taking time to talk as a family. Family-prompted internal meetings are common (Wittenberg-Lyles, Goldsmith, Demiris, et al., 2012). Unlike Manager and Carrier caregivers who often need assistance structuring family discussions to make decisions, the Partner caregiver is often involved in family meetings before meeting with the healthcare team or immediately following a meeting with a healthcare team. While Manager caregivers are quick to make decisions in the meeting with a physician, Partner caregivers typically do not make decisions within these meetings. Rather, Partner caregivers engage in the decision-making process with other family members, which includes addressing conflict related to decision-making within the family (Wittenberg-Lyles, Goldsmith, Oliver, et al., 2012). *Darius* describes his family process in caring for his father with Alzheimer's disease:

> There was a meeting recently we had because his dementia seemed to be getting worse. I'm there for the meeting because I'm the one who sees him every day. After that meeting my siblings and I talk without my dad present to sort of discuss what the next steps will be. I always share my opinions, I'm his caretaker.

Box 7.4

PARTNER DESCRIPTIONS OF UNIFIED FAMILY APPROACH TO
DECISION-MAKING (2019 DATA COLLECTIONS)

- *We talk about it as a family, but always do what the doctor thinks would be best.* (Cancer patient, son caregiver)
- *We always sit down and listen to what the doctor has to say and once he finishes explaining we'll talk about it amongst ourselves. But in the end the decision is always up to her. We just kind of discuss the options back and forth and then it goes from there.* (Congestive heart failure patient, granddaughter caregiver)
- *We usually talk about it as a family, what we think is best, however we trust the doctors. The doctors are doing their job. They are trained. Usually we take their recommendation and go with it. We aren't going to do anything crazy here but we usually trust our doctors and go with what they say.* (Type 2 diabetes patient, daughter caregiver)
- *We talk it over between family members and all try to come to an agreement on a decision.* (Cancer patient, sister caregiver)
- *We make it together, talking out the pros and cons and sometimes my mom's sister will give her input too.* (Cancer patient, son caregiver)

In this case, the family meeting does not include the care recipient as persons with Alzheimer's disease are often not able to participate in decision-making. The same is true for *Adriana*, a 60-year-old Hispanic woman caring for her mother with Alzheimer's disease:

> Together we would make the decision [about treatment]. My siblings and I will make the decision. Not any individual one would do it. We share information, we share what we have seen. We keep notes about what we see, what we do with her, or what she is doing, or anything that is different, and we keep, we share our notes with each other. So, I think, just that our family meetings, we just share what we have.

However, a defining aspect of family decision-making for the Partner caregiver and family members is the recognition and commitment to letting the care recipient make the final decision. Family members share in the process by being present for discussions with physicians, asking questions, reminding the care recipient about questions to ask, and by discussing benefits and drawbacks of options presented. While family members have opinions on what the best option is for their family member, and these opinions are shared, LOW/WARM conformity patterns place priority on autonomy and ultimately serve to preserve and prioritize the care recipient's decision. The Partner caregiver embraces and honors this decision, as illustrated in examples in Box 7.5.

In addition to the proclivity to trust doctors, the Partner caregiver has expectations for communication with physicians and the healthcare team. These expectations include a respectful and relational demeanor towards the caregiver.

Box 7.5

Partner Descriptions of Unified Family Approach to Decision-Making (2019 Data Collections)

- *Typically, I give my opinion to my dad and I normally try to get in the position of what is best for him because I tend to know him a little better so I give him my opinion but ultimately, he makes the decision, but sometimes, I will admit sometimes my decisions have influenced his decision but for the most part he's the one that has the final word.* (Cancer patient, son caregiver)
- *I think the final decision would be hers but for the most part is collaborative. I prefer the patient to make the decision and we always talk about the pros and cons. I think we are very open on respecting my mother's wishes so if this is something she decided after reviewing the pros and cons then we respect that.* (Cancer and type 2 diabetes patient, daughter caregiver)
- *So, after the family meeting my mom was discussing the possible options for which surgery to do and it seemed like everyone had good feedback for her to decide. So, it was a very pleasant meeting.* (Cancer patient, daughter caregiver)

Esme, caring for her mother with breast cancer, shares the difficulty of the doctor–caregiver relationship she has experienced:

> I haven't been asked how I'm doing as a caregiver or what I would want for the patient. My mom's process has been very difficult. We actually had like a lot of complications with her primary doctor in the beginning. The doctor didn't really want people to go in with my mother. He questioned the people that were going into his office with her. . . . It hasn't gotten any easier. . . . There's supposed to be a professional relationship between a doctor and a patient . . . like personal connection, to make the situation go a lot smoother, and make the patient and the caregiver feel more comfortable. And I feel like I haven't really gotten that. I haven't, haven't felt really comforted or felt a sense of relief with the relationship with the doctor.

Armed with these expectations, the Partner caregiver's communication approach with the healthcare team is to be direct.

Carlos is a 28-year-old Hispanic man caring for his mother with an aggressive type of brain cancer. His sister, two brothers, father, stepdad, and sister-in-law all participate in his mother's care, which has included two craniotomies, chemotherapy, and radiation over the last two years. He describes how his communication approach with physicians evolved into a direct approach:

> I feel like I'm more aggressive to make a point or make a comment just because I feel like they don't think I'll have any questions. So, I always kind of like wait, pause, can we reiterate, and then, so just to summarize, because every time the doctor would show us [magnetic resonance images] he'd be like yeah this is how it looks and this is how it looks now, and I'd be like ok so is this better or this worse? So I'll always be more aggressive and try to ask questions.

The Partner caregiver's direct communication approach conveys a comfortableness in working with healthcare providers. Being comfortable in communicating with the care team also enables the Partner caregiver to be proactive in caregiving, where the Manager and Carrier caregiver tend to be reactive.

FAMILY UNCERTAINTY

Partner caregivers face the illness alongside the patient and share the experience of living with uncertainty (Reigada et al., 2015). For the Partner caregiver, uncertainty is related to hope and hope is not seen as a black-and-white option pitted against despair; hope is considered a delicate balance between managing day-to-day symptom management and maintaining a sliver of quality of life (Coelho et al., 2019). *Paco,* whose grandfather is hospitalized for end-stage kidney failure, explains how family members stay focused on maintaining his dignity:

We have a big family, there is seven of us, and the way we were communicating was, who's seeing him, and who's with him. Who's sleeping with him. If you can't make it, if someone has to be somewhere, who can fill in? Because my grandfather can't do much and can only speak Spanish so we want to at least translate for him, or be there for him to give us a request, an uncomfortable request that he might feel shy to ask the nurse.

Whereas Manager and Carrier caregivers are driven by fear of the uncertainty of the chronic illness and the uncertainty of their ability to carry out their role as caregiver in a successful manner that meets their own as well as family expectations, the Partner caregiver's fear is secondary to their desire to the meet the needs of the care recipient. Because their goal in caregiving is to make sure the care recipient's wishes are fulfilled and that quality of life and living is met on a daily basis, their uncertainty remains focused on the care recipient.

While the uncertainty of illness can cause caregivers to hide the painful aspects of caregiving or avoiding communication about illness (Coelho et al., 2019), the Partner caregiver actively communicates about anticipatory grief. Anticipatory grief is present for the Partner caregiver and can include focusing on the day-to-day interactions with the care recipient, grieving for the person they were, and simultaneously beginning to live and plan for life without them in the future (Bouchal et al., 2015). Individuals with high conversation-oriented families are more likely to routinely assess and regulate their emotions (Jones et al., 2017). For the Partner caregiver, heavy reliance on open communication about illness reduces the traumatic distress associated with witnessing suffering, feeling incompetent, and being unable to manage care demands. Partner caregivers take an "approach orientation" to chronic illness, which allows them to acknowledge the impact on the family system and make it controllable by employing social support both within and outside of the family (Coelho et al., 2019).

CONSIDERING PALLIATIVE CARE COMMUNICATION AND HEALTH LITERACY

A seemingly competent and well-organized family structure is in place for the Partner caregiver who naturally serves as family caregiver to the care recipient. A LOW/WARM conformity pattern depicts a close caregiver–care recipient relationship, and family function and decisions are about how best to honor this high-quality relationship and equally care for the caregiver as well as the care recipient. The foundation of this family is a HIGH/WARM conversation pattern depicted by frequent and spontaneous communication about almost any topic related to illness. The ultimate goal of family efforts is to respect the wishes of the care recipient, regardless of conflicting view points, and to recognize and release the stressful role of the caregiver.

The warm communication patterns of Partner caregivers do not exempt them from an isolated illness journey where communication about illness is entirely absent. Despite warm communication patterns that support open awareness of illness, the Partner caregiver can experience high family functioning where illness is discussed within the family but lacks outside communication with healthcare providers. With little information or limited access to information about disease progression, the Partner caregiver and family can get lost in an isolated journey. Resources can be utilized but not maximized. Internally, the family may know that the care recipient's illness is progressing, but if discussions about care remain linear and discretely focused on biomedical aspects by the healthcare team, the Partner caregiver will continue to experience high-functioning family support in the absence of direction from healthcare providers. Overall, their high trust in healthcare providers leaves them with the weakest understanding of the healthcare system among all types (Wittenberg et al., 2019).

The shift to a rescued journey occurs for the Partner caregiver when hospice is introduced. Uniquely, the Partner caregiver and family does not need to be rescued by a healthcare provider who introduces hospice. The HIGH/WARM conversation pattern of this family allows hospice and end-of-life care to be introduced by a provider, another family member or friend, or the Partner caregiver herself. Among all caregiving types, the Partner caregiver is most likely to engage in talk about death and dying with the care recipient (Wittenberg, Kravits, et al., 2017). When hospice is introduced as an available resource that benefits the family (Wittenberg-Lyles & Thompson, 2006), this closely aligns with the goal of the Partner caregiver (in contrast, this would not be an acceptable approach for a Carrier caregiver). Whether or not the family shifts to care that includes end of life care depends on the care recipient, as a LOW/WARM conformity pattern prioritizes the care recipient's decisions above all else. When the care recipient has accepted the disease and can engage in conversations about end of life, the Partner caregiver does not struggle against this and uncertainty segues into anticipatory mourning that can be shared openly. The loss of patient ability to communicate and the supportive role of the patient in making decisions creates a rescued journey for Partner caregivers. As hospice enters, the rescue harbingers anticipatory grief and loss.

The Partner caregiver's direct communication style with healthcare providers, where they or a member of their family will initiate or be open to talking about the end of the disease trajectory, increases the likelihood of a comforted journey that involves palliative care. The Partner caregiver does not shy away from learning as much as possible and information-seeking is driven by a desire to know everything. Unlike the Carrier caregiver who never feels prepared enough for caregiving, the Partner caregiver feels most prepared and is likely to report no unmet needs (Wittenberg, Kravits, et al., 2017). As described previously, the goal of information gathering is to share information with the care recipient to assist with making decisions. This includes initiating topics about prognosis, the future, and quality of life with healthcare providers, even when healthcare providers may not be comfortable discussing these topics. When providers are vague or ambivalent in discussing the course of disease, the Partner caregiver pushes for candid conversations about prognosis.

Since the Partner caregivers' goal is to gain full understanding of the disease, including end of life, their role often includes being responsible for the continuity of care, and their own information-seeking can lead to palliative care (Reigada et al., 2015):

> The last family meeting that we had was when I suggested we start palliative care. Palliative care is when you try to just focus on easing the pain of the patient, getting them ready to head towards hospice. . . . So, I have read about and I suggested it to my family and we all sat down with a palliative care team and they really described what palliative care was to all of us and asked us all our opinions. . . . Everybody had input.

Because family decision-making occurs on its own for the Partner caregiver as part of family coping and adjustment, the Partner caregiver relies on LOW/WARM conversation patterns to find the courage to discuss end-of-life care.

Vital to the success of a comforted journey is that the Partner caregiver does not necessarily serve as the communication hub for the family. Illness information can come from any family member, and Partner caregivers are often given information from other trusted family members. A HIGH/WARM conversation pattern strengthens family resilience and thus benefits collaborative family adaptation to palliative care (Kim et al., 2018). *Isabella* whose mother has had lifelong diabetes and about five years ago was diagnosed with cancer explains how talk about the disease evolved for her family:

> She did receive treatment initially when she was diagnosed but moving forward she opted to not continue her treatment, so right now we are more in a monitoring stage. . . . I think culture wise it would probably be a "hush hush" situation meaning we probably wouldn't talk about it much but over time we've started talking more about her disease and her condition.

Isabella acknowledges that cultural beliefs would have emphasized a HIGH/COLD communication pattern where communication about illness is avoided or ignored, setting the family on an isolated (no end of life care) or rescued (late hospice) journey.

As family communication is expanded to include talk about her mother's condition, the introduction of palliative care and later hospice sets the course for a comforted journey that includes palliative care. In family systems with a Partner caregiver, family members may engage in talk about death and dying with the care recipient, even before circumstances require these conversations (Wittenberg, Kravits, et al., 2017). This is the case for Isabella and her family:

I think we are all aware of what her wishes are. . . . Believe it or not my mother has been very open on letting us know what she wants for whenever that day arrives [dying]. This morning she came in telling me all she wants for the day she passes and what song she wanted to be played. So yeah, it's not taboo; we are super open on that idea, and I'm really blessed because we have that open communication that we are able to discuss those things. We are so lucky that we even get to talk about it. She's aware of what will happen if she doesn't continue her treatment and she's already made up her mind.

The Partner caregiver's role eases as communication facilitates understanding about the disease and support from within the family system. Advance care planning is either in process or in place and discussions about death and dying, while difficult, can be broached within the family system (Wittenberg, Kravits, et al., 2017).

The quality of the relationship between care recipient and Partner caregiver influences how each of them adjusts to chronic illness (Kayser et al., 2018). When the care recipient is vague or ambivalent, the Partner caregiver honors his or her process yet still feels compelled to be prepared for end of life. *Mai* describes the awareness she has about the difference between her own understanding and her mother's understanding of the course of disease:

She's very optimistic and unrealistic at the same time. She's very hopeful. . . . I don't want to take too much away from her so I just let her think what she thinks. Just let her be and treat her with love. . . . It's just about being realistic . . . so this way I can plan accordingly. . . . I'm capable but later on I don't know. I know eventually I'm gonna need help. I've been thinking about that. I might need to talk with some sort of social worker or somebody who will, help me figure all this stuff out because I have no idea. I do need help. Everybody needs help.

It is this steadfast approach to caregiving that propels the Partner caregiver into a comforted journey that involves palliative care during chronic disease management.

SELF-CARE AND THE PARTNER

One of the most unique features of Partner caregivers is their ability to engage in collaborative coping with the care recipient and to also engage in self-care. Partner caregivers have the highest social support and self-care among all caregiving types (Wittenberg et al., 2019) and are least likely to hide opinions about caregiving from other family members (Wittenberg, Kravits, et al., 2017). A LOW/WARM conversation pattern about illness makes it permissible for caregivers to share caregiver burden, which also contributes to their awareness and understanding about the need for self-care. Mai shares how she became aware of the need for self-care:

Sometimes when I go on like two to three hours sleep, for whatever reason and I just, I get irritated. Not at her, just about not having enough time. For nothing. And then I would just have a mental breakdown where I would pray and meditate, talk to a friend, go out and have a little quiet time for myself. Even like an hour or two I've noticed just to be by myself and relax my mind and body. For a while there I wasn't doing that and I, I felt, I was poisoning myself in so many ways and try to take care of Mom at the same time, that was crazy. But now I'm learning how to step back and just make note. That was, that was big for me. That was big. Ever since I've been doing that, things are much better now. I felt like I was just dying. Just, you know, mentally, physically just dying. And come up from air. Now I try to make a little time.

Recognizing that her fatigue has critically impacted her own life, Mai describes not only becoming aware of the need for self-care but also that fatigue has impacted her ability to serve as caregiver. There is room for this awareness for Partner caregivers who can give themselves permission to seek rest from caregiving.

LOW/WARM conversation patterns also positively influence family coping. When family members can make meaning together, vis-à-vis open communication about illness, they are better able to support each other. Open communication about illness does not always come easily, despite the Partner caregiver's LOW/WARM conversation pattern. Mai initially worked hard at convincing her mother to accept her lung cancer diagnosis:

We have disagreement because of, basically I took the, a bunch of information from the American Cancer Society and Natural Cancer Society. And then try to explain to my mom and then I would try to have her even watch YouTube, so she could be aware of what she's dealing with. But she refused and that was big. She's just like, "Nope." I'm putting it right in front of your face, just open your eyes, "Just listen, mom." She don't want it. That was tough, that's very tough. I feel like I'm, I'm doing this the whole battle on my front. She needs . . . to be involved. I feel like she would get something out of it but that was tough to swallow. It's just tug of war. Tug of war. That was the biggest thing though was just communicating at the beginning because at the end of the day, I gotta see her as a sick person. [but] we grew, . . . the biggest part is, I mean it's, this thing has really brought Mom and I together, you know, on so many different fronts.

Mai's efforts to share knowledge with her mother initially failed (and are reminiscent of the Manager caregiver's communication style!); however, a LOW/WARM conformity pattern for the Partner caregiver also means respecting the patient's right not to know or understand. Respecting the patient's decisions and working to ensure patient dignity are defining qualities that separate the Partner caregiver from other caregiving types. This positive family communication process increases family adaptation for the Partner caregiver (Kim et al., 2018), and dyadic coping supports patients' mental health (Lyons et al., 2016).

Relationship quality between caregiver and care recipient uniquely contribute to open communication that enables the Partner caregiver to explore their purpose in caregiving, which also leads to greater caregiving rewards for the caregiver (Polenick et al., 2018). Subjective or perceived burden is the evaluation of stressors in caregiving and are strongly related with caregiver health indicators (Del-Pino-Casado et al., 2018). Caregivers who are securely attached in a close relationship with the care recipient, wherein the two individuals can share their emotions with each other, yields a more positive caregiving experience (Monin & Schulz, 2010). Caregiver burden is minimized by open discussions about caregiver stress (Wittenberg, Buller, et al., 2017). Among all caregiving types, the Partner caregiver reports the lowest distress and the highest quality of life (Wittenberg, Kravits, et al., 2017).

Although the care recipient actively serves as a major part of the Partner caregiver's social support network, one of the struggles for the Partner caregiver is the loss of the care recipient as a source of social support (Wittenberg-Lyles et al., 2013). The relationship quality between Partner caregiver–care recipient has been characterized by open communication; as the care recipient becomes no longer able to participate in decision-making, the Partner caregiver is no longer able to rely on the one person who served as the steadfast support in life. The emotional support once sustained through the relationship is now unreliable, leaving Partner caregivers with a lack of confidence. This is especially salient for Partner caregivers of persons with Alzheimer's disease or dementia as disease progression prevents shared decision-making, which was once a major component of the relationship.

SUMMARY

A LOW/WARM conformity pattern coupled with a HIGH/WARM conversation pattern produces positive family learning for the Partner caregiver, with family members working on their own to adapt, cooperate with each other, and engage in emotions associated with caregiving. (Anderson & White, 2018). Recognized as central to the care of the patient, the Partner caregiver is prioritized within the family system by others who contribute only what they can and when they can, yet support is abundant. The focus is not on preparation as it is for the Manager caregiver, and it is not on family preservation, as it is for the Carrier caregiver. For the Partner caregiver, this togetherness creates a pyramid of care that places the focus on an already high-quality relationship with the care recipient and facilitates high cognitive restructuring, which decreases emotional distress (Palacio et al., 2018). Partner caregivers present to others as *supporter of the experiences of the care recipient* and have the best overall health outcomes, which are likely the result of family adaptation to caregiving (Bouchard et al., 2019). Box 7.6 summarizes the Partner caregiver across the topics explored in this chapter.

Box 7.6

Family Communication Pattern
- Conformity—Low, Warm
- Conversation—High, Warm
- Caregiver experiences influx of family communication but not necessarily family presence

Behaviors in the Illness Process
- Presents to others as *supporter of the experiences of the care recipient*

Family Expectations for Caregiving
- Inherently natural pressure from within self to serve as caregiver, due to relational closeness with care recipient

Family Roles
- Caregiving is team effort, no expectation for caregiver to lead
- Chronic illness is family topic, end of life is acceptable topic
- Caregiving role complements patient role
- Engages in direct emotional support to patient

Family Decision-Making
- Make decision as a family
- Family debriefing after family meeting, internal meetings
- Commitment to care recipient as final decision maker
- Direct communication approach with healthcare team

Family Uncertainty
- Desire to know everything and share with care recipient
- Hope for quality of life
- Anticipatory grief/loss acknowledged

Palliative Care Communication and Health Literacy Considerations
- High family functioning requires direction by healthcare providers
- High trust in providers
- Weakest understanding of healthcare system
- Caregiver shares all information with care recipient
- Information-seeking can include palliative care and hospice

Self-Care
- Collaborative coping with care recipient
- Family coping through open communication
- Caregiver explores purpose in caregiving

REFERENCES

Anderson, E. W., & White, K. M. (2018). "This is what family does": The family experience of caring for serious illness. *American Journal of Hospice & Palliative Care*, *35*(2), 348–354. https://doi.org/10.1177/1049909117709251

Bangerter, L. R., Liu, Y., & Zarit, S. H. (2019). Longitudinal trajectories of subjective care stressors: The role of personal, dyadic, and family resources. *Aging & Mental Health*, *23*(2), 255–262. https://doi.org/10.1080/13607863.2017.1402292

Bouchal, S. R., Rallison, L., Moules, N. J., & Sinclair, S. (2015). Holding on and letting go: Families' experiences of anticipatory mourning in terminal cancer. *OMEGA: Journal of Death and Dying*, *72*(1), 42–68.

Bouchard, K., Greenman, P. S., Pipe, A., Johnson, S. M., & Tulloch, H. (2019). Reducing caregiver distress and cardiovascular risk: A focus on caregiver–patient relationship quality. *Canadian Journal of Cardiology*, *35*(10), 1409–1411. https://doi.org/10.1016/j.cjca.2019.05.007

Coelho, A., de Brito, M., Teixeira, P., Frade, P., Barros, L., & Barbosa, A. (2019). Family caregivers' anticipatory grief: A conceptual framework for understanding its multiple challenges. *Qualitative Health Research*, *30*(5), 693–703. https://doi.org/10.1177/1049732319873330

Colquhoun, A., Moses, J., & Offord, R. (2019). Experiences of loss and relationship quality in couples living with dementia. *Dementia (London)*, *18*(6), 2158–2172. https://doi.org/10.1177/1471301217744597

Conway, E. R., Watson, B., Tatangelo, G., & McCabe, M. (2018). Is it all bleak? A systematic review of factors contributing to relationship change in dementia. *International Psychogeriatrics*, *30*(11), 1619–1637. https://doi.org/10.1017/S1041610218000303

Del-Pino-Casado, R., Frias-Osuna, A., Palomino-Moral, P. A., Ruzafa-Martinez, M., & Ramos-Morcillo, A. J. (2018). Social support and subjective burden in caregivers of adults and older adults: A meta-analysis. *PLoS One*, *13*(1), e0189874. https://doi.org/10.1371/journal.pone.0189874

Hou, W. K., Lau, K. M., Shum, T. C. Y., Cheng, A. C. K., & Lee, T. M. C. (2018). Do concordances of social support and relationship quality predict psychological distress and well-being of cancer patients and caregivers? *European Journal of Cancer Care (Engl)*, *27*(4), e12857. https://doi.org/10.1111/ecc.12857

Jen, C.-H., Chen, W.-W., & Wu, C.-W. (2019). Flexible mindset in the family: Filial piety, cognitive flexibility, and general mental health. *Journal of Social and Personal Relationships*, *36*(6), 1715–1730.

Jones, S., Bodie, G., & Koerner, A. (2017). Connections between family communication patterns, person-centered message evaluations, and emotion regulation strategies. *Human Communication Research*, *43*, 237–255.

Kayser, K., Acquati, C., Reese, J. B., Mark, K., Wittmann, D., & Karam, E. (2018). A systematic review of dyadic studies examining relationship quality in couples facing colorectal cancer together. *Psycho-Oncology*, *27*(1), 13–21. https://doi.org/10.1002/pon.4339

Kim, G. M., Lim, J. Y., Kim, E. J., & Kim, S. S. (2018). A model of adaptation for families of elderly patients with dementia: Focusing on family resilience. *Aging & Mental Health*, *22*(10), 1295–1303. https://doi.org/10.1080/13607863.2017.1354972

Lyons, K. S., Miller, L. M., & McCarthy, M. J. (2016). The roles of dyadic appraisal and coping in couples with lung cancer. *Journal of Family Nursing*, *22*(4), 493–514. https://doi.org/10.1177/1074840716675976

Monin, J. K., & Schulz, R. (2010). The effects of suffering in chronically ill older adults on the health and well-being of family members involved in their care: The role of emotion-related processes. *GeroPsychiatric Nurse (Bern)*, *23*(4), 207–213. https://doi.org/10.1024/1662-9647/a000024

Palacio, C., Krikorian, A., & Limonero, J. T. (2018). The influence of psychological factors on the burden of caregivers of patients with advanced cancer: Resiliency and caregiver burden. *Palliative & Supportive Care*, *16*(3), 269–277. https://doi.org/10.1017/S1478951517000268

Polenick, C. A., Sherman, C. W., Birditt, K. S., Zarit, S. H., & Kales, H. C. (2018). Purpose in life among family care partners managing dementia: Linking to caregiving gains. *Gerontologist*, *59*(5), e424–432.

Reblin, M., Stanley, N. B., Galligan, A., Reed, D., & Quinn, G. P. (2019). Family dynamics in young adult cancer caregiving: "It should be teamwork." *Journal of Psychosocial Oncology*, *37*(4), 526–540. https://doi.org/10.1080/07347332.2018.1563582

Reigada, C., Pais-Ribeiro, J., Novellas, A., & Gonçalves, E. (2015). The caregiver role in palliative care: A systematic review of the literature. *Health Care Current Reviews*, *3*(2), 143. https://doi.org/10.4172/2375-4273.1000143

Wittenberg, E., Buller, H., Ferrell, B., Koczywas, M., & Borneman, T. (2017). Understanding family caregiver communication to provide family-centered cancer care. *Seminars in Oncology Nursing*, *33*(5), 507–516. https://doi.org/10.1016/j.soncn.2017.09.001

Wittenberg, E., Goldsmith, J. V., & Kerr, A. M. (2019). Variation in health literacy among family caregiver communication types. *Psychooncology*. https://doi.org/10.1002/pon.5204

Wittenberg, E., Kravits, K., Goldsmith, J., Ferrell, B., & Fujinami, R. (2017). Validation of a model of family caregiver communication types and related caregiver outcomes. *Palliative & Supportive Care*, *15*(1), 3–11. https://doi.org/10.1017/S1478951516000109

Wittenberg-Lyles, E., Goldsmith, J., Demiris, G., Oliver, D. P., & Stone, J. (2012). The impact of family communication patterns on hospice family caregivers: A new typology. *Journal of Hospice & Palliative Nursing*, *14*(1), 25–33. https://doi.org/10.1097/NJH.0b013e318233114b

Wittenberg-Lyles, E., Goldsmith, J., Oliver, D. P., Demiris, G., & Rankin, A. (2012). Targeting communication interventions to decrease caregiver burden. *Seminars in Oncology Nursing*, *28*(4), 262–270. https://doi.org/10.1016/j.soncn.2012.09.009

Wittenberg-Lyles, E., Washington, K., Demiris, G., Oliver, D. P., & Shaunfield, S. (2013). Understanding social support burden among family caregivers. *Health Communication*, *29*(9), 901–910. https://doi.org/10.1080/10410236.2013.815111

Wittenberg-Lyles, E. M., & Thompson, S. (2006). Understanding enrollment conversations: The role of the hospice admissions representative. *American Journal of Hospice & Palliative Care*, *23*(4), 317–322. https://doi.org/10.1177/1049909106289077

Zhang, Y. (2018). Family functioning in the context of an adult family member with illness: A concept analysis. *Journal of Clinical Nursing*, *27*(15–16), 3205–3224. https://doi.org/10.1111/jocn.14500

Spotlight

Navigating

One of the overarching difficulties for caregivers who are caring for a family member long term is discovering how to navigate the current complexities of the U.S. medical system. As Arthur Kleinman (2019) describes in his recent book chronicling his own caregiving experiences with his wife who suffered from early onset Alzheimer's, patients and family members are involved in a constant state of "waiting" when one is seriously ill: This waiting—for diagnosis, for appointments, for test results, for doctors' follow-up calls—exacerbates the stress of being ill. Prolonged waiting communicates to patients and family caregivers that they are mechanistic cogs in the vast machinery of medicine, that healthcare providers see a patient as one more set of symptoms to diagnose, one more body to be scheduled for service.

The difficulties and protraction of wresting a diagnosis can cause profound stress for patient and caregiver alike. Likewise, uncaring doctors at the time of diagnosis create added anxiety: Lucy spoke of a doctor who told her and her husband, immediately after he was diagnosed with Lewy body dementia, "Get your affairs in order because in one year you won't even recognize who you are." Caregivers quickly discover that they must bear most of the burden of discovering where to locate the best care for their loved one. Those with health literacy skills and resources (see Chapter 2 of this volume) know how to search for renowned clinics and physicians. Those endowed with resources are able to visit the best clinics in the country and to see the best doctors for second and third diagnostic opinions and for state-of-the-art treatment options.

Frequently, family caregivers are the ones who must locate clinical trials and assess their goodness of fit. Lucy described the frustration of trying to speak to the administrators of various trials who never returned her calls and of numerous trips to enroll in a trial. Money and time and persistence were required; she was unsure whether her husband would have pursued the clinical trial option had she not insisted on it. Attempting to understand the language of the protocol of a clinical trial proved almost impossible, even for PhD-educated friends whom she consulted. Health literacy in this context appeared unattainable! Once accepted and enrolled in a trial, visits to its host clinic, three hours away, were frequent and burdensome. Yet being in the trial proved an enjoyable experience since its medical personnel "seem to care about their patients." Concern expressed for the patient and the integrity of the staff helped ameliorate the disruption to their lives that constant travel created. Still, Lucy questioned whether choosing to participate in a clinical trial was the right path: She feared that they might be missing a limited opportunity to travel to places they loved because of commitment to the trial. The uncertainty of Chuck's disease progression made her second-guess every major decision.

For Carolina who was caring for Waldo in his final months, coordinating the nonfamily caregivers was her most difficult caregiving task. Although Carolina was herself a retired nurse, she was shocked by the physical challenges of caregiving and needed professional caregivers to assist her with overwhelming physical tasks. As Waldo became sicker and weaker, moving him and getting him from Point A to Point B was a major dilemma for her. Especially when he became bedbound, Carolina was forced to hire help. But hiring, "training," and monitoring agency caregivers gave her major headaches: "Not all caregivers are created equal" was her constant refrain. Paid caregivers were not always trained to do basic caregiving activities such as changing diapers, giving bed baths, changing bed linens, and turning patients to avoid bedsores. Carolina had to be the trainer in many cases, but not all paid caregivers were willing learners! She felt that someone in the family had to monitor the professional caregivers if she couldn't be at home to do so herself: She did not feel that Waldo was safe otherwise. Further, she experienced incidents of caregivers stealing money from the home, even while family members were present. It was galling to Carolina that one caregiver let Waldo sit in wet clothing for many hours without offering him a urinal or taking him to the bathroom. The need to constantly monitor hired caregivers made Carolina feel tethered to her home since she felt complete responsibility for the care Waldo received there. This did not make her want to place Waldo in institutional care—she was proud of the care she gave him at home and felt that it was a way of demonstrating her love and devotion to him, but her 24/7 sense of being responsible did add significantly to her caregiver burden.

Managing both the professional care of their loved one—from visiting various MD experts and enrolling in and traveling to clinical trials—and also managing nonfamily, professional caregivers attached significant burden to family carers' intrinsic and weighty caregiving tasks. Although family caregivers may not express resentment about these management responsibilities since they are willingly sought, they do readily admit to the added stress, money, time, and energy such tasks entail.

8

The Lone Caregiver

It's a huge burden. All of a sudden, I've gone from being a wife to a complete caregiver and managing all the medicines and the driving. These tests come up in your mind about "how sick is he?" Is he okay to do this? Do I have to be careful about this? Is it okay for him to drive? But he is still the same man. I have to stop looking for signs. It doesn't mean oops, there he goes, this is it. The slide begins. He doesn't have the memory that he did. He doesn't have the cognitive abilities. It doesn't mean that he is diving down. Some days it feels like everything is on a downhill slope and I don't want to be the last person standing.

—Lucy, former teacher, wife of Chuck

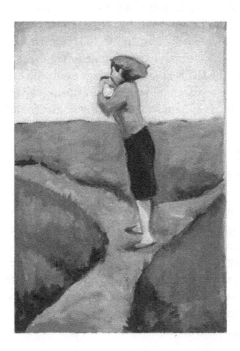

The caregiver illustrated in this chapter illustration depicts a person having to choose a path. For the Lone caregiver, in particular, the navigation of the path is punctuated by extreme solitude during the journey in ways that the other caregiver types are not. A tension is infused into this painting and suggests risk and loss in a precarious environment—a place where anything could happen. Anything could go wrong or right. And the decision made by the caregiver may determine that outcome. The Manager and Carrier paintings also present a solitary figure encountering a struggle. All of the figures are active and doing something difficult in each illustration. But it is *what* and *how* they are accomplishing that action that resonated with our writing team's typology and the particular caregiver type they represent. The figure is focused not on the pushing and pulling or balancing of a task. Rather the caregiver's focus is sent to decision-making to act—to select the best road to travel. The stakes feel very high and can impact life or death.

We feature two Lone caregivers in this chapter (Lucy and Viv Gray), and along with their stories, we weave in additional narrative experiences from a range of Lone caregivers from across the country. Lucy, aged 68, lives in South Texas with Chuck, her 65-year-old husband of 18 years. A second marriage for both of them produced a blended but very distant family. Two years ago, Chuck, a whiz with any technology or engineering feat, began struggling with sequencing. After an odyssey of physicians and diagnostics, Chuck was diagnosed with Lewy body dementia. This is his only chronic illness, unlike the story of Viv and Jake Gray.

Unlike Chuck's single, chronic illness diagnosis, Jake was living with multiple comorbidities, some of which were still not clearly diagnosed and only identified under the umbrella term of Gulf War illness. Yet each man's circumstance communicates the complexities of struggle in chronic illness for the caregiver. Although only in his late 40s, Jake's physical and psychological illnesses had aged and disabled him beyond his years. Chronic pain and fatigue took shape after his deployment to Iraq in 1991. Living with acute posttraumatic stress disorder (PTSD) and its array of maladies was the driving ailment for him and Viv, but in the last year Jake was diagnosed with type 2 diabetes. A 50-pound weight gain in a year, total wakefulness during the nighttime hours, and a fragmented healthcare system have complicated care for all of his life-limiting challenges.

NAMING THE LONE CAREGIVER

The early English term "all one" serves as the root of the term *lone*, and it denotes the state of being apart from others. For the purposes of the caregiver typology, the "others" this caregiver is apart from are family members and their potential network of support (Oxford English Dictionary, 2019). The name of this Lone caregiver has always been different than the other three names. As we have tried to be clear in this volume about the strengths and weaknesses of each type, we want to start the conversation about the Lone caregiver by looking at parts of speech. The Manager, Partner, and Carrier—these are all nouns. It may seem that we have singled out the Lone caregiver by giving it the classification of an adjective. Here is our opportunity to describe that naming more thoroughly than we have had the chance to do prior.

The term *lone* is one that is observable in culture, and underscoring its use in some specific contexts may help flesh out our understanding of this caregiver type. The Lone Ranger, an enduring iconic American character, first depicted in radio and then film and television, is the only survivor of an ambushed group of Texas Rangers. The Lone Ranger fights for justice, is an expert marksman and orienteerer, is unique in his approach to negotiating powerful forces, is industrious with resources and ideas, and manages these gifts in solitude—apart from a group.

The Lone Wolf has become a common phrase/concept in Western culture that is derived from the stealth of this beautiful animal, the wolf, normally a pack animal. Either resulting from purposeful exclusion from a group or choosing solitude, the wolf has been observed with some frequency to do things on its own—preferring to be an individualist, nonconformist. The phrase has been integrated into literature and culture—often describing characters who are individualists, serious, and somewhat reserved in nature and who operate independently and stealthily. Replacing some of the potentially pejorative implications of this caregiver's title with other language and cultural references makes more room to describe this particular caregiver's strengths and needs.

FAMILY COMMUNICATION PATTERNS OF THE LONE CAREGIVER

Lone caregivers represent approximately 15% of the caregivers we have studied during the last decade. This group experiences very limited or nonexistent family support as a result of low family conformity and conversation. Caregivers who have limited support from within their social network (family and friends) endure high strain throughout chronic illness and end of life and represent the most compromised and burdened subpopulation of caregivers (Lee & Robert, 2018). Without a substantive family or network of support, this caregiver experiences oppressive burden resulting from intensive caregiving. Although caregiving research has received a great deal of attention, a paucity of knowledge regarding these most isolated caregivers leaves a void of evidence to inform appropriate caregiver education and intervention. We describe this Lone caregiver as a person who is in a constellation of family but is not receiving regular or engaged caregiving support from the family. In fact, this caregiver may even live across the street from family or see family members while at the grocery or drug store—but it is not a family that operates in an environment of regular communication or expectations of conformity.

The Lone caregiver exists in a communication climate of LOW conformity in addition to low conversation. The dimension of conformity establishes and protects hierarchies and structures in a family. Group harmony and the protection of roles are not important or prioritized in families with low conformity. The family roles and structures are not central or protected in family communication. So, as the Lone caregiver emerges from a context of low conformity, this conformity can also be classified as COLD. COLD conformity is demonstrated through a lack of consistency in family rules, sharing beliefs that demonstrate inequity, not recognizing protected family times/rituals, and avoiding the cultivation of family closeness (Hesse et al., 2017). Because of the low component to conformity, this caregiver is unaccustomed to fixed structures around shared family responsibility and events, does not participate with family members to create opportunities to remain connected, and is not engaged in communication that expresses family values centered on closeness (Hesse et al., 2017). Taken together, the dimensions of LOW/COLD conformity serve to define the environment of interaction for the Lone caregiver family structures and hierarchies.

The dimension of conversation is low for the Lone caregiver, who experiences very infrequent conversation among family members. The conversational interaction is typically nonspontaneous when it does occur, and if a spontaneous interaction does take place it is typically because of an unplanned sighting in a public space. Low conversation patterns decrease opportunities for families to discuss illness, dying, death, and planning ahead for exigencies of illness.

We extend the WARM/COLD description into the dimension of conversation and observe the Lone caregiver as experiencing COLD conversation (Hesse et al., 2017). The missing or nonexistent expectation of agreement and assimilation in conversational topics establish conversation as a COLD theoretical classification. There is no requirement to express agreement and alignment, and as a result, this family experiences difference and distance in their interactions, and the action of conversation itself confirms the remoteness that the Lone caregiver experiences in the family. The family's uncoordinated patterns of interaction engineer the incongruous nature of the interaction itself. Little is accomplished or processed when communication does take place. Accounting for both dimensions of the communication environment allows us to name the Lone caregiver as LOW/COLD in conversation.

The Lone caregiver navigates a stealthy and resourced journey of care. Speed and swift action are far less important than exploring every best opportunity for increased physical recovery and maintenance for the care recipient. Exercising rigor in knowing health information and possible places of care drive this caregiver's work and burden. Navigation, orientation, and execution—these are three areas of preoccupation as the Lone caregiver seeks, finds, acquires, and receives medical support from systems and providers for the care recipient's illness(es).

Without an integrated family system of expectations to negotiate, the Lone caregiver can discern the care process without the burden of involved additional parties advocating for differing positions and ideas. Similarly, a streamlining of care may be the result of this unified caregiver effort. Without multiple responsible players in the caregiving mix, there is a perhaps a less conflicted journey of care in the family.

This caregiver primarily communicates with others about the physical needs and requirements of the patient, and this becomes the center of the caregiving labor. The psychosocial needs of the patient remain more peripheral to the Lone caregiver's efforts. The care recipient's needs, behaviors, and opinions about health information and decisions are important in the work of the Lone caregiver. The two may disagree or treat aspects of care very differently, but the Lone caregiver is highly keen to observe the position of the care recipient concerning their values around the illness(es). The Lone caregiver readily moves forward on a course of care without family support for that journey.

LONE BEHAVIORS IN THE ILLNESS PROCESS

The onset of illness marks the entry into caregiving. Acute onset is sudden, with minimal time for planning or reflection. The Lone caregiver does not have family mobilization and acts with resourceful and thorough efforts to position the care recipient to receive the best physical care. Seeking best care is the point of focus for this caregiver. Researching, communicating, and pursuing are central in this period. A protection of the care recipient is an element during this time, but not to the exclusion of communication about care and decisions with the care recipient. There can be a frenetic aspect to the Lone caregiver's labors in acute onset, but it is important to know that researching and pursuing are significant elements to this work. Making care choices is the goal, but not for the sake of just having a plan. It has to be the plan that will be the most effective. Lucy describes the onset of Chuck's illness and the haunting indicators that his mental functions were changing. In her narrative, she reveals her keen observations of his changing behaviors, but also the painful communication with a provider.

I knew something was wrong because he was having trouble sequencing things. He's always been the TV person, and he would know how to operate all the TV things. And he was forgetting how to do that. And I knew at that point something was wrong. He had two other symptoms that are very characteristic. He was seeing dogs in the corners of his eyes. This had been going on for like three or four years. We thought it was refractions from his glasses, so we replaced them. We would joke about what kind of dog it was, and then he would see a cat. These were hallucinations. In fact, not long ago he told me that sometimes there's a third person in the house. So the hallucinations are one thing, but then there is also an REM sleep disorder, which is prototypical. He jumps out of bed. He hit a piece of furniture and broke a window. He talks in his sleep, and kicks. He used to hit me and that's when we decided we better go to a sleep therapist. When we went back to the sleep doctor with a diagnosis from the neurologist, the doctor said, "I suggest you get all your affairs in order because next year you won't even know who you are."

In gradual illness onset, the Lone caregiver acts as a very close monitor of mounting and patterned signs of illness of the care recipient. Without a family system to engage in the caregiving journey, the Lone caregiver relies on the healthcare system stakeholders for information and interaction regarding care decisions. Gathering facts about treatment approaches and illness process are important to this caregiver. For this caregiver, psychosocial provisions for the care receiver do not receive the same attention that biomedical management receives. There is a dependence on healthcare providers to fill the gaps that family network planning and decisions accomplish for other caregiver types. But in the end, the Lone caregiver adheres most regularly to care plans and navigates care with greater skill than the other types.

Navigating care resources, piloting the illness and its progress with the care receiver, and pursuing physical improvement are earmarks of the Lone caregiver. This caregiver is outside the support structure of a family and may or may not be able to offer hands-on physical care consistently and over time that other types might more readily achieve. Therefore, the Lone caregiver and their care recipient are a unit of care decision-making and management and sometimes work very closely as a team in the tasks surrounding care and its decisions. The Lone caregiver presents to others as *seeking the most effective physical relief and support* for the care recipient and performs this role in interactions shared with others. An awareness of the care recipient's ongoing physical loss and struggle is evident in communication with the Lone caregiver, as a well as a driving desire to implement care that will alleviate a patient's pain, deficits, and losses. This caregiver is sure to identify what is helping, what would help, and what they (i.e., patient/caregiver) hope will help. There is not only a desire to manage the unmanageable nature of chronic illness progression, but also a trepidation for the impending changes ahead. A desire to control the forward movement of the illness process is expressed and enacted by the Lone caregiver. Concern about the losses ahead are at the fore of their discussions with others, as well as an expressed urgency to make changes or implement care plans that are possible.

To add some further understanding about the Lone caregiver, we include simplified aspects from Julian Rotter's theory of locus of control. Rotter proposed that some of us live life with an *internal* locus of control and connect actions with outcomes. Another way to think of this might be to connect pursuit and action with results. Those with an internal locus of control believe that the outcomes of their actions are results of their own abilities. Internals believe that their hard work will lead them to obtain positive outcomes. In short, actions produce effects. Opposite this framework is the *external* locus of control, which includes people who believe that events that occur are outside what an individual can impact and a result of external elements like the power of others, fate, luck, mystery, etc. A multifaceted and textured set of causes move the responsibility and control of events outside the person with an external locus of control (Rotter, 1966).

These two oppositional approaches to believing in our actions and the powerful forces outside us are not two separate ideas. Rather, Rotter intended for the two loci to live on a continuum where individuals could identify their tendencies

(Rotter, 1966). And those tendencies change as life changes. As adults experience more health challenges and events, they tend to believe less and less that their own actions may be impacting what is happening to their bodies (Jacobs-Lawson et al., 2011). We mention this continuum of locus of control because the Lone caregiver's strongest intention is to impact the physical quality of life of their care recipient. Controlling the physical is very important to this caregiver. But this doesn't mean that the Lone caregiver does not experience an external locus of control. As diseases advances and more physical challenges arise, the impact of personal behaviors and actions are less understandable and explainable. The Lone caregiver focuses on seeking solutions and improvements from a clear biomedical position, as demonstrated by our caregiver voices throughout this chapter. Because of the reduced impact of family conformity and communication, the Lone caregiver is not only able to independently pursue physical care without familial conflict or negotiation, but also must take this task on without substantive social networks established through the family system.

In the course of the illness(es), the level of intensity in caregiving will undoubtedly vary. The Lone caregiver primarily experiences care as one acute crisis event after another, forming a fixation on the physical aspects of illness and dying. The Lone caregiver gauges the level of activity and labor around the physical well-being of the care recipient. Periods of lighter caregiving are welcome opportunities to recover from manic efforts to manage the physical challenges of side effects and disease advancement. Seeking out new health systems, treatments, and providers occupies this caregiver across all periods of care. The Lone caregiver arranges appointments and all that goes with that, including transportation, housing, food, and respite care. Because of their need to create a network of support outside the family structure, the Lone caregiver and care recipient have the unique burden of figuring everything out and dealing with it. We have learned from studying the Lone caregiver that this burden may in some cases be less onerous than navigating the demands and presence of family support. We can see this focus on the physical in Lucy's description of seeking a clinical trial for Chuck's Lewy body dementia.

I mean I had to push for that. [Research hospital] never called me back. They have some issues with their phone system. I would leave a message. I called all the time; it didn't come easily. And then we had to drive over there. They don't take people in the clinical trial that weren't their patients. So Chuck had to become their patient. So we had to go over there, and he had to go through, become a patient, and then we had another time to go over there to make sure he was qualified for the clinical trial. And then the third time they accepted that. So it was not an easy process. All of these steps require money, and fortunately we could afford it. And just persistence, which is where I came in. I don't know if Chuck would have done it by himself. Probably not. And so that's where you're [the caregiver] pushing. But I couldn't live with myself if I didn't. If it's out there and it's a possibility, right. And then you can always say, well, I was altruistic even though he personally didn't benefit. . . . I love him. I want to keep him alive. That's my primary, my primary goal and we want to keep him healthy.

Lucy describes her motives. At the core, she articulates her fear that she would regret not trying every path on behalf of Chuck. All stones would be unturned to make his journey the least painful one. You can also hear the solitary nature of her navigations. Lone caregivers are isolated from family. Their interaction and decision-making about healthcare takes place in and around the healthcare system; they seek out support beyond the family to inform their decision-making. These are targeted pursuits. For Lucy, the path to the clinical trial also included a close examination of documents that informed her decision on behalf of Chuck. She sought out people in her circle to help interpret language and think through potential complications in committing to a trial. The healthcare professionals were the other set of teammates she relied on. For the Lone caregiver, families surrounding the patient are distant and uninvolved, even if they are nearby. Caregivers like Lucy and Viv know *a lot* about places of care and providers and are heavily focused on the biomedical fires in their midst. The psychosocial elements of chronic illness fall well behind the physical worries for this caregiver. There is a sense in listening to Lone caregivers that a remedy to make things better is there. It exists. But it is not yet found. At the same time, the remedy is not necessarily thought to be a cure-all, but rather as a way to make the physical costs less severe, less painful, and less burdensome to the care recipient.

The primary support and decision-making relationships outside the Lone caregiver and care recipient are those shared with healthcare professionals. Most of their shared healthcare interactions will address the physical needs of the patient. Topic content; subject matter; and goals of care conversations exchanged between the Lone caregiver, the care recipient, and healthcare professionals center on the physical needs, symptoms, side effects, and disease path. This caregiver designs and plans the next barrage of attacks on the illness by capitalizing on biomedical action. The rub can quickly become the care recipient, who may or may not align with the Lone caregiver's level of demand. Lucy has learned that vigorous and frequent exercise is a measure that will slow the progression of Chuck's illness. She describes desperately wanting for Chuck to enact a vigorous plan of exercise to stave off the advancement of Lewy bodies.

It's been a huge bone of contention. All of our marriage and now that I feel like he could be managing this disease by working out because with Lewy body comes Parkinson's, and one of the ways you treat Parkinson's, and I know this because of my sister, is that you work out feverishly about five to six days a week for 45 minutes to an hour. It's been proven that yes, because blood flow to your brain, if you think about it. It's working out like that at a continued rate of speed with your heartbeat at a particular level is very helpful. I don't see him doing that. He will when he gets on the elliptical. He does get on the elliptical. He also goes to physical therapy. He goes to physical therapy twice a week. They stopped that for a while. They had to get approval. So he's in the interim doing his thing with a personal trainer. So he's doing things, but at home he sits, and I don't think that's healthy.

For Lucy, it is irrational to do anything other than everything. And to the reader (and to the authors), it appears that Chuck *is* doing a great deal. He is using an elliptical at home, has physical therapy, and is responding to Lucy's plan by working with a personal trainer in the interim.

For the Lone caregiver, part of the ceaseless search for biomedical healing is the abiding *hope* in what medicine offers. This caregiver type believes and follows the path of cure and the narrative of restoration, in so far as it fits (Goldsmith et al., 2016).

The Lone caregiver is often unaccompanied by others for appointments. Because of their lone status, their work is done in the company of the care recipient. What could be mistaken for a defensive exterior of mistrust with healthcare professionals may also be described as a quest for treatment. Their focus on the biomedical needs of the care receiver is primary, which at once leads them to rely heavily on the medical system for caregiving, support and guidance.

In Viv's Words: Chasing

I know that he could be better. And we are chasing so many things at one time with his health. With every change in medicine, there is a great impact on the side effects we experience. He is taking so many things and changing one thing shifts the others. Last count was 14 scripts taken throughout the day. I feel like we can do better. I feel like we haven't really tackled the core of the challenges, which is the Gulf War illness. I think that anyway. I think he believes that too. But we are pretty fatigued from chasing all of it. The diabetes probably wouldn't be on the table if the sleep were straight, and the psych meds were less. But no one person is really willing to look at the whole picture. And so it's like we are always chasing pieces. Just making to an appointment, even if it is a telehealth appointment, is a huge challenge. I end up rescheduling a ton of them. On a day when there is an appointment so many things have to line up for us—starting with the night before, which is really his day. His primary physician at the VA [Veterans Affairs] said to me, "His sleep needs to get straightened out immediately." She is clueless. Completely. She has no idea of the theater of war he participated in, or the earmarks of acute PTSD. So how do we navigate that? The VA doesn't get it. How can she work in the VA system and be completely unaware of night terrors and related anxiety? So all of this spins and piles us, and the type 2 goes out of control.

Viv centers her worry on one dimension of his care—his physical status and the convoluted, multifaceted difficulties of his physical health. This is representative of the Lone caregivers we have studied. Communication and effort are focused on problem-solving across physical quality of life challenges much more so than psychosocial aspects of care (Wittenberg-Lyles, Goldsmith, Demiris, et al., 2012). Viv recognizes the primary difficulty accompanying Jake's PTSD, but seeks to manage it primarily through pharmaceuticals. Since the Lone caregiver relies on healthcare staff to navigate and execute care, there could be frequent opportunities to engage this caregiver in interactions about quality-of-life concerns—not only for the care recipient but also for the caregiver. But in Viv's case, the healthcare system represents a missed opportunity to engage in psychosocial support. Viv's story allows us to see the role of the system in caregiver burden. As seen in Box 8.1, lone caregivers share their experience with and reliance on the healthcare system and healthcare team when communicating and understanding the care recipient's medical regimens.

Lone caregivers described the benefits of and desires to receive one-on-one communication from team members as well as specifically framed questions and conversations that are about the caregiver, not simply the patient. They described these two communication practices as the conduit to team involvement and belongingness (Wittenberg-Lyles, Goldsmith, et al., 2012a). These findings align with similar caregiver research concerning team communication (Skorpen Tarberg et al., 2019) and the positive benefits of individual attention from team members.

FAMILY EXPECTATIONS AND ROLES

In the family system, the Lone caregiver experiences low or noninvolvement with low or no interference from family in and around the illness context as a result of their LOW/COLD conformity and communication patterns. This can be a gift

---

Box 8.1

LONE CAREGIVERS DESCRIBING MEDICAL ASPECTS OF CARE (2019 DATA COLLECTION)

- *I think when she is in pain that's the time to take medicine. Everybody's worried about if they get addicted, or you know . . . if you should take your medicine. That's the least of their worries, you know.* (Cancer patient, daughter caregiver)
- *How can I leave him, you know, for—even for three or four days like that? If he gets a fever or chills, uh, I have to monitor him, and take him to a doctor, or call for him because we got nobody else that we can count on for him.* (Cancer patient, son-in-law caregiver)

LONE CAREGIVER PERCEIVED COMMUNICATION WITH PROVIDERS (2019 DATA COLLECTION)

- *Don't get me wrong, I am well aware of the fact that you're talking about the patient. Sometimes maybe you need to talk to the caregiver.* (Cancer patient, sister caregiver)
- *I feel that they are too busy or something. Even the information sometimes— that I don't get enough information. But it's like there's no explanation. They just say a few words, and then that's it.* (Dementia patient, daughter caregiver)

---

as well as a barrier to caregiving relief. But the family system that exists without demands of conformity or conversation does not shift to increase either communication component due to illness. The system is the system and remains so in the face of health challenges. This caregiver is not positioned to rely on family or receive support that may address caregiver burden. The Lone caregiver does not expect or initiate a different experience with family based on these very long-standing patterns in the communication environment (Wittenberg-Lyles, Goldsmith, et al., 2012b) as illustrated in Box 8.2. The family type that produces the Lone caregiver also includes a flexibility that caregivers from high-conformity environments do not offer (Wittenberg-Lyles, Goldsmith, Demiris et al., 2012).

Communication within the Family

His sister came over and she was talking about me searching for solutions and she said, "You're pushing into so many things [treatment options]." She said if the roles were reversed Chuck wouldn't be doing that.
                                        —Lucy describing a conversation with Chuck's sister

Because the Lone caregiver has LOW/COLD conformity and communication and the lowest family conformity and conversation dynamics of the four caregiver types, it makes sense that research reveals their sharing about medical appointments, health news, and all other conversation subjects are also at the lowest rate (Wittenberg, Kravits, et al., 2017). In accord with the low rates of interaction, Lone caregivers indicate the lowest percentage across all

---

Box 8.2

Lone Descriptions of Family Expectations (2019 Data Collections)

- *We have other family, but none that supported either one of us.* (Cancer patient, son caregiver)
- *He has a sister that lives, uh, close—well, not that close by, but not that far away, like only about maybe 10 miles away. I tried to tell his sister—call him—"He's sick," and something like that because I know that they kind of—they got along. Then something happened. So when I call to tell her, because, the point that I want to make is that if she wants to talk to him or something like that, I can kind of try to bring them together. Maybe go between here and there or something because we don't know if he'll be able to meet with her, talk to her, ah, later on, you know? And because they're brother and sister, I know that he loves his sister. I know that, you know, brother and sister have, you know—I know that for me, I love my brother and sister, so I expect people maybe are like that, too. But then, when I call her, it's like—she said she has her own problems.* (Cancer patient, son-in-law caregiver)

---

of the caregivers in experiencing unmet needs in the family. The expectation of support and shared burden is simply not present for this caregiver as it is with higher conformity family systems like the Manager and Carrier. In fact, the enmeshment that is very much a part of high conformity systems increases caregiver burden. Since the occasion to interact or seek agreement is so rare, the Lone caregiver is less encumbered with this communication labor of achieving family harmony in the face of family illness stressors as illustrated in Box 8.3.

Having low family support requires the Lone caregiver to seek support networks to cope throughout the caregiving experience. Those caregivers with low familial support networks are more likely to use counseling, respite, and other resources to aid in coping. In the same study, caregivers who reported a low social network had higher preference ratings for support services compared to caregivers with high social networks (Lee & Robert, 2018).

In Viv's Words: It's the Two of Us
I don't think my family really has a clue. Occasionally they ask about us, and about him. And mostly express their amazement at how difficult his care sounds. But they usually don't ask. His mom does stay in touch. It seems like we have settled on a once a week text that arrives from her usually on the weekend with a report from her world. And that's nice. But we are truly alone. His sister lives with his mom. There's just no togetherness. His kids are young and several states away. Somehow his world is so small. And it seems like my world is him.

With the family distant in shared communication, the caregiver and care receiver's private information surrounding illness is less a negotiated factor.

Box 8.3

LONE COMMUNICATION WITHIN THE FAMILY (2019 DATA COLLECTION)

- *They don't care about him, especially his father. He never cared. And the youngest one lives in Washington. It seems like he doesn't care much. He either calls his father on the phone and talks in there, but, he doesn't care much. The bottom line, his family—my father-in-law's family, only, I care for him. The rest of it seem like—with his wife, his two sons, they, they, like, you know, it's like they try to stay away from the, uh, problem (inaudible) and anything like that.* (Cancer patient, son-in-law caregiver)
- *My family left me alone to care for my Mother. If it were not for Larry, I don't think I could do it. Because my brother gives no care whatsoever, he hasn't even been to see Mom. He could get here, he's retired, he could be here.* (COPD patient, son caregiver)

Communication privacy management (CPM) and ownership of knowledge about the illness is the most limited for the Lone caregiver when compared to other caregiver types and, in essence, is a less onerous burden (Venetis et al., 2014). Additionally, the stakes for sharing information and the impact of that sharing with family may be less weighty, as the expectations for interaction and family values are far less a factor. Family may learn of private information by being told by a person close to the Lone caregiver or through social media and less commonly by the Lone caregiver or care recipient themselves.

Communication with the Care Recipient

Another sign of lower communication burden for the Lone caregiver is their more open communication with the care recipient. Together they share information about the disease and its treatment and talk together about interactions with healthcare professionals (Wittenberg, Borneman, et al., 2017). The Lone caregiver shares a unique relational resource in the care recipient because of the relatively minimal family network of support. The emphasis placed on the dyad of caregiver and care recipient impacts disclosure or concealment communication behaviors between the two. Concealment behaviors mask distressing information directly or indirectly related to a care receiver's medical condition. Self-concealment increases psychological distress (Wertheim et al., 2018) as the concealer is tasked with covering and withholding distress that may be essential for making decisions and identifying goals.

The companion to self-concealment is perspective taking. If personal information is shared, then the other part of the dyad has the chance to perform perspective taking, which puts one person in the other person's shoes and demonstrate shared concern (Wertheim et al., 2018). Thinking of concealment on a continuum may help us understand the Lone caregiver burden further, as there are some relationships that are dependent on concealment and some that are not, and the range of those that fall in between.

It makes sense to look closely at the communication between the caregiver and the care recipient in particular, as we seek to understand the Lone caregiver and discern the specific communication practices that can increase or relieve caregiver burden. Sharing in the illness appraisal as well as collaborating in the management of illness is sometimes undertaken as communal coping between the caregiver and care receiver. Discussing illness-related issues; combining efforts, skills, and knowledge to engage in joint problem-solving; and negotiating responsibilities establish a set of communication behaviors that involves both caregiver and receiver in addressing illness-related issues (VanVleet & Helgeson, 2019). Communal coping occurs when individuals hold a shared appraisal of the illness and also collaborate in illness management. This communal coping may occur most especially for the Lone caregiver and care receiver, as social support for them often is defined by the support they provide for the other as described in examples in Box 8.4.

Box 8.4

LONE COMMUNICATION WITH THE CARE RECIPIENT (2019 DATA COLLECTION)

- *I talk with her to see what she actually wants to do. So, we talk about it.* (Diabetic patient, niece caregiver)
- *We just sit and talk about it and go from there.* (Diabetic patient, daughter caregiver)
- *Then my father-in-law said he didn't want to go through the treatment. I said, "You have to go through it because your doctor that wants to help you, and then you don't go through. What do you think your grandson's going to think about you?" That's how he feel like, you know? So I try to encourage him, but all at the same time, try to, you know, like, make him feel like—to be strong and, and don't be weak, you know. I know that he's scared, but then, uh, even at this time, too, I feel like maybe he doesn't want to go through with it. Yesterday he mentioned to me that, you know, he doesn't know if he can last—like, go through the whole chemo series.* (Cancer patient, son-in-law caregiver)
- *I tell him that he needs to know, so basically, I don't hide from him if (inaudible) if it's going to hurt him, if it's going to make him feel sad (inaudible) it's the truth, I tell him.* (Cancer patient, son-in-law caregiver)
- *The end of life decision, no. I, I never talk to him about that. We talk about the treatment only. I want to talk to him about that, too, but, you know, uh—I have not talked to him about it. And also, I don't know if he wants to talk about it, you know? Sometime people might not want to talk about end of life. And I wanted to—basically, I wanted to, like, ask him, you know, what is his wishes, something like that, if it—if he passes away? Like what kind of funeral does he want?* (Heart failure patient, niece caregiver)

In Viv's Words: Together

It has to be okay with him, or we won't do it. But whatever it is—I put that together. I am always ready to cancel or change an appointment. I have to be. Pressure will not help his outcome. I am committed to caring for him, not to my plans and schedules for him. Some days we can go for help. Other days, we need to just let him rest in bed. The pain is the devil and dictates his sleep. It's very hard. I couldn't ever have imagined doing this. But I also can't imagine doing life without him.

This grouping of narratives from Lone caregivers further demonstrates the challenge of goal multiplicity. The care recipient and caregiver will often hold differing goals and even multiple goals—some realized and some still unrealized to each individual (Tracy & Coupland, 1990). Depending on the dyad, these multiple goals are negotiated sometimes with more ease than for other dyads. Because communicators pursue multiple and often competing goals, problems and dilemmas can be common in interaction, and for the Lone caregiver their care recipient is at times their primary collaborator in navigating illness. The instrumental goals of the Lone caregiver can dominate, as care treatment and solutions to pain and progression are pursued. But we can readily read in the voices of these caregivers that there is always a competing set of goals that speak to their relationship and trust as goals are revised and rewritten.

DECISION-MAKING AND UNCERTAINTY

This caregiver's primary interlocutor in decision-making about care and how it will be pursued is the care recipient. This is a unique identifier of the Lone caregiver. The care recipient figures prominently as a decision-making for the Carrier, and also as a focal point for the larger family in the Manager and Partner caregivers. But for the Lone caregiver, there is no populated family system that serves to weigh in, agree, disagree, challenge or convolute the caregiving decisions. The main player who serves to bring dimension and multiple perspectives to care decisions is the care recipient. Lucy describes decision-making differences between her and Chuck that she has to deal with.

> Our personalities are as different as they can be. I do everything today. Chuck? [He] is "What's the rush?" What's the incentive? He gets things done.... He's not a procrastinator. He was a very successful businessman. But when it comes to other things like fixing something that he could probably do, what's the big rush? It a huge, been a huge bone of contention. All of our marriage and not that I feel like he could be minimizing this disease by working out. . . . Chuck is much more sedentary than I am, and now it's becoming more difficult to see him do that because I feel like he's losing. He needs to be fighting harder. . . . He gets resentful that I push. He doesn't get resentful that I leave. I hack at him. I'm a great nagger. I can be a very mean aggressive woman and I can be, and I say things that I'm always ashamed of saying, and I'm always apologizing for it. So for somebody that has a nature, like I do, this push and aggressive fight in me, I don't know any other way of doing it. We're very different in that regard. In other ways we're very much alike. The loss of somebody that you absolutely adore is something else. I don't want to go through that. I think I can do it [care for a debilitated Chuck]. I think I will do it because I care for him that much. But then you want to pull back parts and part of you wants to pull back and say, I need to preserve myself. We hold hands in bed. We sit on the sofa next to each other. I mean, it's a very very sweet relationship. Many people don't ever get that. I am really very very grateful for that. I ask my therapist, 'Will I ever be happy

again?' And I have these moments of great happiness and joy when I see Chuck doing well. When he does something that's the least bit [worrisome], cause you look for stuff. "Oh, here it [dementia] comes." You look for failure in them.

Lucy is suffering because of their push–pull over differences in how they pursue care. She describes their conflict from the standpoint of her regret over communication choices she has made in talking with Chuck about his care. Lucy is ready to act and be aggressive with his treatment. Chuck is not accommodating her demands. And Lucy suffers guilt and regret for demanding he align with her preferences and exhibiting such harshness.

Maybe I'm too intense, maybe I'm too intense about this [Chuck's care]. Where do you draw the line? I don't know that. I don't know where to draw the line. I'm letting it [finding care for Chuck] cause me anxiety. I need to back off and let Chuck make some decisions. All that uncertainty. . . . It's his life. It's not my life. I can't impose my life or the way I would do it on him. I have to back off. . . . I'm not going to be one of those women that never leaves their home that waits on their husband hand and foot. I can't do it. I don't want to be like that.

Lucy verbalizes her struggle with wanting Chuck to do what she wants him to do to minimize his illness and letting Chuck be who he in this illness. She is articulating exactly the negotiation of her own *multiple goals*—help him and Lucy live better longer or lay down that goal and replace it with grace. It is impossible to separate the relational and task duality here, as is so often the case for caregiving decisions and actions.

CONSIDERING PALLIATIVE CARE COMMUNICATION AND HEALTH LITERACY

As a result of our most recent studies exploring the caregiver typology, we have assembled new knowledge about health literacy and how it relates to caregiver communication and burden. We learned about the ways that caregiver communication patterns influence their ability to locate, access, and trust resources and information. In our early work, some assumptions about the Lone caregiver left us wondering about their health literacy skills since they were solitary actors outside of a family who could support the caregiving effort. Could they be in a more difficult position to find, understand, and communicate about health information and decisions than those caregivers who are surrounded by family support and labor? The answer is generally *no*. The Lone caregiver most often has high skills and abilities than the other three caregiver types concerning health literacy.

Remember our description of Lone in the early part of the chapter—excellent at orientation and negotiation, nonconformist, and individualist? This caregiver is keen on knowing the services available, the roles of people in a given healthcare setting, and the hierarchies in the healthcare context; the Lone caregiver is the independent navigator primarily negotiating shared decisions with the patient. The Lone caregiver may challenge providers as a result of their own ardent research and careful investigations. In fact, a care provider may misinterpret the caregiver's tenacity and direction resulting from careful planning and investigation as obstinacy.

In Viv's Words: VA Health Literacy
Every day I check his VA portal. Sometimes I have written notes to his provider team; other times I am checking his prescriptions to see what should be ordered or picked up, and sometimes I look for resources because they are changing so often. The real bummer though is that not all of the appointments and services are findable on the portal. That's where we fall through the cracks. He may have received calls or emails, but I haven't. I am not the patient. Does the VA really think that 80-year old vets are checking their phones? Let alone the 40-year old disabled ones? It doesn't all line up. The wheels really come off when we have appointments that are outsourced to community care—which is what happens when the VA can't handle the load. Those appointments never appear on the portal. So, sometimes I wonder if the portal can get any less useful.

An analysis of caregiver types and their health literacy related to communication with providers, care recipient, and knowledge of the healthcare system demonstrated that the Lone caregiver has the highest functioning knowledge of the system (Wittenberg et al., 2019). Their proclivity to navigate independently and cultivate a pathway of care in conjunction with the care recipient correlates with a high level of health literacy. This recent research adds dimension to our understanding of communication patterns and the caregiver's ability to locate and access care for the recipient. Select examples of Lone caregiver health literacy descriptions are listed in Box 8.5 below. In Chapter 2 of this volume, we described the features of health literacy and how it is a construct achieved through the abilities of every stakeholder. Some of those stakeholder roles are integrated into the words of the caregivers in Box 8.5.

In Viv's Words: Health Literacy Meets Real Life
I love Jake. It wasn't until I moved in with him that I understood the enormity of caring for hi, and how that would affect every part of our life. He has been disabled for almost a decade, because of sleep and PTSD, which has now created extensive weight gain issues and eating challenges leading to his type 2. His driving is intermittent. There are days when driving for him is not an option because of anxiety. And me driving is a definite no. We have tried

Box 8.5.

LONE CAREGIVER DESCRIPTIONS ABOUT HEALTH LITERACY (2019 DATA COLLECTION)

- *She can't speak English. She only speaks Korean, so whenever she goes to the hospital, I have to translate for us. And she doesn't understand still.* (Diabetic patient, granddaughter caregiver)
- *In the United States you have to make appointments in advance. And then you won't get seen by your doctor for months. In Korea, you can go every single day and get care.* (Diabetic patient, granddaughter caregiver)
- *We have a high belief in homemade remedies so that is always part of the conversation.* (diabetic patient, daughter caregiver)
- *I get all the information and relay what I feel is necessary back to my daughter [7-years of age] . . . in simpler terms.* (Diabetic patient, mother caregiver)

that. One day he almost dove out of the passenger side of the car because of panic. Here's an example of one of my daily challenges. Sometimes I can't get inside our house. I leave for work, and he has to use both locks on the inside in order to feel like he can actually sleep. My key only opens the deadbolt from the outside. When I come home, usually around 3:00 in the afternoon, he is still asleep—actually just entering into his fifth or sixth hour of sleep. I will call his phone to let me in. But about half of the time he doesn't hear it. The phone is a major issue. He misses about five calls a day from the VA. These calls are for appointments. The VA policy will not include me on these calls, only the patient. So it is truly hit or miss. If he thinks to go through the messages, or send them to me, we can calendar his appointments or re-schedule them. About half of the time that doesn't happen, and the system has us start back at the beginning of the line to make an appointment with a specialist, like the endocrinologist.

How does our new knowledge about the Lone caregiver intersect with the three potential illness journeys of isolated, rescued, and comforted? We see these three pathways as so heavily dependent on the providers and systems available to the care-giver that potentially any of the three are possible. The strong preponderance of the Lone caregiver to pursue biomedical concerns could readily invite the pathway of the isolated journey, if there are no participating voices incorporating other aspects of emotional, mental, and social care into the range of concerns for this caregiver.

SELF-CARE AND THE LONE CAREGIVER

There is now plentiful evidence that connects caregiver burden to compromised physical and social health for the caregiver. Additionally, compromised health for the caregiver leads to less positive patient outcomes. Specifically, caregivers facing long-term caregiving tasks involving multiple areas of need experience increased depression and anxiety adapting to the caregiving role, dealing with uncertainty about the future, and enduring a lack of support across social networks (Woodford et al., 2018).

> Chuck says I'm killing myself. He has a geriatrician that tells me the same thing. She can tell when I go in with Chuck and she sees my anxiety and how much I worry, and she says, "We have to deal with you. Your husband's doing fine." I'm hoping there's some spiritual benefit from caring for someone you really, really, love and that it compensates for the loneliness that you feel, and for the isolation and the sadness; that giving to someone is a compensation.

The Lone caregiver experiences the lowest level of self-care. This corresponds to this caregiver's lack of social support. While the low-conformity family structure removes some of the decision-making conflict and stress from this caregiver, there is also decreased opportunity to find time to leave the care recipient alone and attend to their own healthcare, social needs, and financial demands. Relief may be very hard for this caregiver to find, as they are truly apart from their family group and must rely on the care recipient, friendships, and healthcare providers for the bulk of their decision-making communication (Wittenberg et al., 2019). Because of minimal family support, this caregiver type is at high risk for caregiver burden. Family caregiving for cancer patients is associated with significant occupational impacts, financial impacts, distress, and other negative health impacts with caregivers having very little time to look after themselves, high rates of depression and anxiety, and low mental health-related quality of life (Lightfoot et al., 2019). The Lone caregiver is at high risk for these woes and rates highest across the caregiver types for quality-of-life distress.

Desired resource support for family caregivers include respite services, care coordinators, telephone support line, consistent policies and procedures, knowledge about hospice, and instrumental support (MacLeod et al., 2012). Lone caregivers are especially in need of help with communication with medical staff and family members, stress management, self-care, emotional support, bereavement care, and resource finding (Kutner et al., 2009). Lucy describes the outside support she is receiving from a therapist to help her navigate anxiety over Chuck's disease, and her vigilance in identifying symptoms and decline.

> This is why I need to go back to the therapist, and I've talked to him [to Chuck] about this at length after our blow up yesterday. I can't blow up at somebody who's got dementia. You can't do that. You don't know if he's doing what he is doing because of exhaustion. Is it part of Lewy body? You get tired. Well, hell, I don't know if it's this, is it fatigue? How can I be doing that to somebody who's tired? I don't know how to draw the line in being a helpmate and the support, and just being shrew. I don't know where that line is.

Lucy describes her distress in so many of the narratives that appear in this chapter. Distress and anxiety are costly concerns that the Lone caregiver experiences. The illness journeys we incorporate in Chapter 1 of this volume (isolated, rescued, comforted) are particularly salient in the discussion of caregiver self-care (Wittenberg-Lyles et al., 2011). The journeys were originally conceptualized to describe health system resources and health communication made available to a patient and caregiver and would determine the journey for that family. What the caregiver receives from providers and systems determines, to large extent, the type of illness journey that the caregiver will experience. We posit that the illness journey for a family caregiver is influenced by (a) the approach to caring for the patient (curative only versus curative/comfort), (b) health literacy of stakeholders, (c) the structure and communication of care, (d) the awareness of the illness and how it is recognized, (e) opportunities to plan for worsening outcomes and end of life, and (f) community versus isolation in care (Witteberg-Lyles et al., 2010). The comforted journey is the pathway we see as the most beneficial for the caregiver. But the self-care embedded in this path cannot be a provision created by the caregiver alone. It is a product of the system and providers surrounding that care receiver and the family communication patterns and caregiver burdens that result.

SUMMARY

Lone caregivers derive from families with low conformity and conversation. Regular exchanges of interaction are not part of their family experience, nor are ritualized dates, behaviors, and times together. The members of this family group are stars in the same constellation, but have no responsibility or time dedicated to one another. LOW/COLD conformity is demonstrated through a lack of consistency in family rules, sharing beliefs that demonstrate inequity, not recognizing protected family times/rituals, and avoiding the cultivation of family closeness (Hesse et al., 2017). LOW/COLD communication is characterized by low expectation for agreement and assimilation in conversational topics and frequency of interaction.

The dyadic dynamic with the care recipient may serve to be its own significant support for some Lone caregivers. These two collaborators, in some care situations, may help share the burdens of decision-making, planning, and even care management. The absence of a family support network moves the Lone caregiver outside of family structures to develop resources and help in caregiving. Healthcare providers and system resources are especially vital in supporting care decisions, goals, and self-care. The Lone caregiver has levels of facility with information seeking and care navigation/pursuit and presents to others as seeking of the most effective physical relief for the care recipient. This caregiver is particularly bound to the care recipient, vigilant about an unfolding disease path, and in high need of self-care resources and respite. Box 8.6 summarizes the Lone caregiver across the topics explored in this chapter.

Box 8.6

Family Communication Pattern
- Conformity—Low, Cold
- Conversation—Low, Cold
- Little to no family network to offer or interfere with care
- Caregiver engages in researching care options and monitoring illness patterns

Behaviors in the Illness Process
- Presents to others as *seeker of the most effective physical relief for the care recipient*

Family Expectations for Caregiving
- No family system support network

Family Roles
- Primary family role is relationship with care recipient
- Other family is minimal in role and support
- Caregiver needs are part of dynamic shared with care recipient

Family Decision-Making
- Make decisions with recipient, with support from providers
- Desire to exhaust any treatments that will slow or stop disease process
- Desire to employ any relief or mediation to physical disease process

Family Uncertainty
- Uncertainty is managed by seeking solutions

Palliative Care Communication and Health Literacy Considerations
- Focus is on physical mediation
- Tendency to experience a rescued or isolated journey due to biomedical focus
- Higher confidence in provider selection
- Higher confidence in place of care

Self-Care
- Very low self-care

REFERENCES

Goldsmith, J., Wittenberg, E., Platt, C. S., Iannarino, N. T., & Reno, J. (2016). Family caregiver communication in oncology: Advancing a typology. *Psycho-Oncology*, *25*(4), 463–470. https://doi.org/10.1002/pon.3862

Hesse, C., Rauscher, E. A., Budesky Goodman, R., & Couvrette, M. A. (2017). Reconceptualizing the role of conformity behaviors in family communication patterns theory. *Journal of Family Communication*, *17*(4), 319–337.

Jacobs-Lawson, J., Weddell, E., & Webb, A. (2011). Predictors of health locus of control in older adults. *Current Psychology*, *30*, 173–183. https://doi.org/10.1007/s12144-011-9108-2

Kutner, J., Kilbourn, K. M., Costenaro, A., Lee, C. A., Nowels, C., Vancura, J. L., . . . Keech, T. E. (2009). Support needs of informal hospice caregivers: A qualitative study. *Journal of Palliative Medicine*, *12*(12), 1101–1104.

Lee, E., & Robert, L. (2018). Between individual and family coping: A decade of theory and research on couples coping with health-related stress. *Journal of Family Theory and Review*, *10*, 141–164. https://doi.org/10.1111/jftr.12252

Lightfoot, N., MacEwan, L., Tufford, L., Holness, D. L., Mayer, C., & Kramer, D. M. (2019). Who cares? The impact on caregivers of suspected mining-related lung cancer. *Current Oncology*, *26*(4), e494–e502. https://doi.org/10.3747/co.26.4635

Lone. (2019). *Oxford English Dictionary*. Retrieved from https://en.oxforddictionaries.com/definition/money

MacLeod, A., Skinner, M. W., & Low, E. (2012). Supporting hospice volunteers and caregivers through community-based participatory research. *Health & Social Care in the Community*, *20*(2), 190–198. https://doi.org/10.1111/j.1365-2524.2011.01030.x

Rotter, J. (1966). Generalized expectancies for internal versus external control of reinforcement. *Psychological Monographs*, *80*(1), 1–28. https://doi.org/10.1037/h0092976

Skorpen Tarberg, A., Kvangarsnes, M., Hole, T., Thrønæs, M., Støve Madssen, T., & Landstad, B. L. (2019). Silent voices: Family caregivers' narratives of involvement in palliative care. *Nursing Open*, *6*, 1446–1454. https://doi.org/10.1002/nop2.344

Tracy, K., & Coupland, N. (1990). Multiple goals in discourse: An overview of issues. *Journal of Language and Social Psychology*, *9*, 1–13.

VanVleet, M., & Helgeson, V. S. (2019). I am a rock; I am an island: Implications of avoidant attachment for communal coping in adults with type 2 diabetes. *Journal of Social and Personal Relationships*, *36*(11–12), 3711–3732. https://doi.org/10.1177/0265407519832671

Venetis, M. K., Magsamen-Conrad, K., Checton, M. G., & Greene, K. (2014). Cancer communication and partner burden: An exploratory study. *Journal of Communication*, *64*, 82–102. https://doi.org/10.1111/jcom.12069

Wertheim, R., Goldzweig, G., Mashiach-Eizenberg, M., Pizem, N., & Shacham-Shmueli, E. (2018). Correlates of concealment behavior among couples coping with cancer: Actor partner model. *Psycho-Oncology*, *27*, 583–589. https://doi.org/10.1002/pon.4552

Witteberg-Lyles, E., Goldsmith, J., Ragan, S. L., & Sanchez-Reilly, S. (2010). *Dying with comfort: Family illness narratives and early palliative care*. Cresskill, NJ: Hampton Press.

Wittenberg, E., Borneman, T., Koczywas, M., Del Ferraro, C., & Ferrell, B. (2017). Cancer communication and family caregiver quality of life. *Behavioral Sciences (Basel)*, 7(1), E12. https://doi.org/10.3390/bs7010012

Wittenberg, E., Goldsmith, J., & Kerr, A. (2019). Variation in health literacy among family caregiver communication types. *Psycho-Oncology*, 28(11), 2181–2187.

Wittenberg, E., Kravits, K., Goldsmith, J., Ferrell, B., & Fujinami, R. (2017). Validation of a model of family caregiver communication types and related caregiver outcomes. *Palliative & Supportive Care*, 15(1), 3–11. https://doi.org/10.1017/S1478951516000109

Wittenberg-Lyles, E., Goldsmith, J., Demiris, G., Oliver, D. P., & Stone, J. (2012). The impact of family communication patterns on hospice family caregivers: A new typology. *Journal of Hospice & Palliative Nursing*, 14(1), 25–33. https://doi.org/10.1097/NJH.0b013e318233114b

Wittenberg-Lyles, E., Goldsmith, J., Parker Oliver, D., Demiris, G., & Rankin, A. (2012a). Targeting communication interventions to decrease oncology family caregiver burden. *Seminars in Oncology Nursing*, 28, 262–270. https://doi.org/10.1016/j.soncn.2012.09.009

Wittenberg-Lyles, E., Goldsmith, J., Parker Oliver, D., Demiris, G., & Rankin, A. (2012b). Targeting communication interventions to decrease caregiver burden. *Seminars in Nursing Oncology*, 28, 262–270.

Wittenberg-Lyles, E., Goldsmith, J., & Ragan, S. (2011). The shift to early palliative care: A typology of illness journeys and the role of nursing. *Clinical Journal of Oncology Nursing*, 15(3), 304–310. https://doi.org/10.1188/11.CJON.304-310

Woodford, J., Farrand, P., Watkins, E. R., & LLewellyn, D. J. (2018). "I don't believe in leading a life of my own, I lead his life": A qualitative investigation of difficulties experienced by informal caregivers of stroke survivors experiencing depressive and anxious symptoms. *Clinical Gerontologist*, 14(4), 293–307. https://doi.org/10.1080/07317115.2017.1363104

Our culture has made us believe that the best care we can give to a loved one is the kind of care that is self-sacrificing, that considers the loved one's interests above all else. Caregivers often feel guilty if their own needs supersede those of their family member's and if they give voice to those needs. Lucy, whose husband has been recently diagnosed with Lewy body dementia, expresses misgivings when she leaves her husband at home to pursue her full, very active social life. Although he currently is stable and in good health, she feels that she needs to stay with him. Yet she also adamantly exclaims "I can't sacrifice myself by never leaving the house", and she also states: "Maybe I'm too intense about this. . . . Where do you draw the line?"

Discovering some balance between caring for the other and caring for oneself is a continual and painful conundrum for caregivers of loved ones with chronic and terminal illness. Lucy expresses a need to pull back, to self-preserve while also wishing to be as good a caregiver for Chuck as she's able to be. When asked what she most fears, Lucy quickly asserts: "I fear most losing Chuck and being stuck at home forever. . . . I can't not go out and not have a life. I can't give up what gives me life." She is concerned about when it will be necessary to enlist paid caregiving help at home or whether she'll have to decide that Chuck needs institutional care. Her friends and her sister warn her that she's already too self-sacrificing.

Carolina, who has been intensively involved in caregiving for Waldo for many months, states that "care is not meant to be 24/7." Trained as a nurse, Carolina is accustomed to long shifts, but caring for a loved one at home means "you're on 24/7." She is exhausted from such a lengthy caregiving stint and says to her husband: "I love you dearly, but understand I need a break . . . and the only thing I want to hear from you is 'have a good time.'" Fortunately, she did hear these words from Waldo! While Carolina has employed professional caregivers to assist her with Waldo's home hospice care, she laments that these caregivers must be constantly monitored since "all paid caregivers are not created equal." Caregiving for her has been an isolating, exhausting task that requires back-up and time for herself. "You're dealing with death every day and you want to feel the rush, you want to feel alive, and this is not, this is you're tethered to someone's bed and to their needs. You have to put everything you want and need aside in order to do this."

Constant caregiving has given Carolina stress reactions so that she designates a two-hour period to rest each day. More important, caregiving has made her miss her personal freedom. She feels tethered and responsible for what goes on in her home. She also misses spending time with her out-of-state family whom she's neglected during her months of caregiving. While she's constantly hosted her husband's family from his first marriage, she has not seen her own. She particularly misses one of her favorite hobbies, reading, and has been unable to focus on books, even when she feels she has a little time to read. Crocheting, making Christmas stockings, pillowcases, and hats for the homeless and the LGBTQ+ community, and sewing afghans have been a diversion for her.

Lucy, whose husband's diagnosis is fairly recent, is also concerned about stress and mental health issues. Taking good care of herself through physical activity, healthy eating, and social connections has always been pivotal to her healthy sense of self, and she's determined to continue this lifestyle. But the anxiety wrought by Chuck's diagnosis has taken a toll: She comments: "Chuck says I'm killing myself worrying," and their geriatrician comments, "We have to deal with you. Your husband's doing fine." She finds herself being quick to anger and constantly apologizing. Yet Lucy is also keen on self-preservation: she sees a therapist and feels that her sessions with him have been helpful. She also engages in constant effort to educate herself about her husband's disease and was pivotal in getting him enrolled in a clinical trial. These proactive activities are mutually beneficial to the couple.

The downside of putting one's life on hold while caring for a loved one is the panic that can ensue of not knowing what to do with your life when your loved one dies. Both Carolina and Lucy have tried to confront this fear: Carolina has written about her plans following Waldo's death: "You should have an idea of what your next step will be." She has also shared some of her ideas with friends. Lucy, anticipating the fear of losing Chuck, has already begun to think about different housing options. She is also determined to maintain her social network and the many activities that give her life meaning apart from Chuck.

9

Caring for the Family Caregiver

We believe that caregiver support must take place from a foundational understanding by healthcare providers regarding the health literacy and communication challenges experienced by family caregivers. We advocate that caring for the family caregiver requires a palliative care communication approach between caregivers and providers to position the caregiver as an essential member of the healthcare team. The Family Caregiver Communication Typology (FCCT) provides a framework for this. While we always advocate for using a health literacy universal precautions approach, the proposed framework will be one more "tool in the healthcare provider toolkit" specifically focused on fostering family caregiver education and support. This chapter offers communication strategies and suggestions for a palliative care communication approach based on caregiver types using a communication and health literacy framework.

As the preceding chapters have demonstrated, there is great variance in communication patterns and health literacy needs among family caregiver communication types. Caregiver assessment should take into consideration the family system and include factors such as lifestyle and behaviors, physical and mental health, social needs and support, health literacy and communication, and lastly, community resources and care coordination needs (Bennett et al., 2018). Caregiving intensity, feelings of appreciation by the care recipient, and caregiver evaluation of interactions with healthcare providers are also important factors to consider (Campione & Zebrak, 2020; Zavagli et al., 2019). There is little evidence for caregiver assessment and interventions based on unique social and contextual factors of caregiving. These deficiencies bring up several challenges for the provision of family-centered care during the chronic illness journey.

CURRENT ONE-SIZE-FITS-ALL APPROACH

First, current approaches to caring for the family caregiver involve a "one size fits all" approach where a primary family caregiver is designated in the medical record and *caregiver assessment may or may not occur*. Most family-centered care models advocate for a universal approach to caregivers and focus on pediatric populations (Kokorelias et al., 2019). While a generalized caregiver assessment provides an understanding of the caregiver's needs, current assessment tools do nothing to understand the reason behind these needs. As the preceding chapters have shown, caregiver needs vary and caregivers place different levels of priority on these needs (Bangerter et al., 2019). Unique caregiving settings produce primary and secondary stressors for caregivers (Gerain & Zech, 2019) and clarity and complexity of content are context specific (Parker & Ratzan, 2019). Caregivers and healthcare providers play different and varying roles that are due to a range of individual and contextual factors (Bucknall et al., 2020).

Second, there is *no link between identification of caregiver needs, recommended resources, and caregiver utilization of resources.* Caregiver assessment is needed to determine appropriate support services and resources needed to ensure high-quality care and to reduce negative caregiving outcomes and improve caregiver satisfaction (Zavagli et al., 2019); however, there remains a disconnect between assessment and the scope and range of resources offered to caregivers. Concerns remain over the amount of time assessment may take as well as how healthcare providers will be able to ascertain appropriate services for individual caregivers (Thomas et al., 2018). For example, changing illness trajectories are not currently included in family-centered care models (Kokorelias et al., 2019).

Third, current caregiver assessments often *do not involve unique caregiving characteristics that positively impact communication and health literacy.* Caregiver characteristics have been identified as set of determinants for caregiver burnout and include background, sociodemographic, psychological, and physical factors (Gerain & Zech, 2019). Little is known about the intrinsic factors that influence caregiver communication during discussions between providers and caregivers (Bucknall et al., 2020). Understanding differences between caregiver types is essential to understanding the influence on the illness journey of the patient and caregiver. Caregivers with less socioeconomic status, fewer resources, and poverty experience more burden and a disadvantaged quality of life (Chappell, 2016). There is a need to account for the social determinants of health for family caregivers, and health literacy is considered a "new" social determinant of health due to its relationship to similar factors (Rowlands et al., 2017). Enhanced health literacy can be a powerful mediator (Logan et al., 2015).

Fourth, current approaches to chronic illness *do not include any resources or training for healthcare providers in how to care for the family caregiver.* Providers do not always know how to engage and involve family caregivers in communication (Bucknall et al., 2020). Communication strategies and illness-specific information for caregivers is currently lacking, leaving healthcare providers with few tools available for implementing family-centered care (Kokorelias et al., 2019). Providers need education that identifies best practices for collaborating with family caregivers (Bell et al., 2019).

AN ALTERNATIVE: CARING FOR THE FAMILY CAREGIVER

The communication needs and characteristics revealed in various ways through the Manager, Carrier, Partner, and Lone caregiver types heighten the need to integrate and teach a palliative care communication approach to chronic illness to care for the family caregiver. A palliative care communication approach may or may not include a palliative care provider but does ensure that conversations about chronic illness include a two-stage, layered awareness where the end of a disease trajectory is acknowledged and an understanding of the factors/ signs of impending death are discussed (Gonella et al., 2019). When structured approaches to include family are missing, there is greater likelihood of an isolated or rescued journey, increasing caregiver burden and leaving family caregivers to initiate topics about disease and the end of the disease trajectory with healthcare providers (Bucknall et al., 2020). To ensure a comforted journey based on open communication and awareness, healthcare providers should engage in a variety of communication strategies to support caregivers and specifically communicate disease-specific information (Kokorelias et al., 2019). Caregiver awareness and understanding of the care recipient's disease trajectory, especially at end-stage or advanced illness, is important to the promotion and acceptance of palliative-oriented care (Gonella et al., 2019).

We offer Caring for the Family Caregiver, a communication and health literacy framework, to assist healthcare providers in a family-centered care approach to chronic illness. The aim of the framework is to enact a palliative care approach to communication by providing tailored clinical practices for healthcare providers and by addressing family caregiver communication types. Using a tailored health communication approach for caring for family caregivers enables healthcare providers to clearly communicate the best available science and evidence-based information and ensure that ethical and cultural contexts of health literacy needs are met (Parker & Ratzan, 2019).

The FCCT provides a tailored approach for caregiver communication and health literacy in the context of the whole family of origin. For healthcare providers, the typology provides a lens for identifying health literacy needs in the context of broader system-level engagement. The FCCT gives healthcare providers a way of assessing and understanding the deficits in caregivers' needs, their priorities, and strategies for how best to introduce appropriate services to meet these needs (Bangerter et al., 2019). In this way, providers can do more than just refer to available local and community resources; they can also identify areas for tailored interventions that address the priorities of caregiver needs as well as the reason for the need. They can also learn how to better use caregiver type information to develop a person-centered treatment plan and how to refer and connect patients and caregivers with available community resources to improve health outcomes (Behforouz et al., 2014).

A silhouette of each of the six framework domains are described next.

Finding Disease Information

Obtaining disease information is an important piece of the caregiving puzzle. Caregivers need to be screened for what type of information they want and how much information they would like. The FCCT demonstrates that caregiver types vary in the type and topic of information caregivers prioritize and find useful (Table 9.1).

Table 9.1. FINDING DISEASE INFORMATION

Recommended Provider Strategies		
• Ask about caregiver main concerns regarding disease • Ask what the caregiver already knows and/or previous experience with disease • Ask how caregiver prefers to find disease information (library, search web, friends, etc.) • Begin disease information discussion with caregiver concerns and priority topics • Review caregiver specific disease information incorporating plain language • Incorporate use of graphics, pictures, models etc. as needed • Provide written disease information for later reference and review • Request caregiver feedback regarding information and resources provided • Suggest reliable resources for additional information • Provide contact information for future questions		
Caregiver Type	***Caregiver Need*** (what this type needs but may not realize)	***Caregiver Preferences*** (what this type is drawn to and receptive of)
Manager	• To find information for clarifying places of care and providers who are available	• Information on disease path • Treatment options and related resources • Descriptions of side effects and symptoms
Carrier	• To find information about hands-on caregiving tasks	• Physical changes for patient • Common reactions to treatment • Physical, social, and cognitive changes for the patient
Partner	• To find information to share with the care recipient and other caregivers for informed decision-making	• Information on disease path • Physical, social, and cognitive changes for the patient • Descriptions of side effects and symptoms
Lone	• To find information about aspects of care that focus on long term goals and social and mental health of care recipient	• Information detailing the range of care options • Information with a focus on physical impact of disease processes • Information that supports preventative measures in care

© Comfort Communication Project

Assessing and Integrating Information

Assisting the caregiver in examining the quality and amount of information that will help them in achieving good patient care is essential (Table 9.2). Interpreting the information with the caregiver is a necessary aspect of working together to

Table 9.2 ASSESSING AND INTEGRATING INFORMATION

Recommended Provider Strategies
- Discuss caregiver specific priorities and concerns (e.g., impact to quality of life—food, sleep, and comfort).
- Describe plan of care and symptom management at home
- Discuss plan for pain management at home
- Collaboratively create caregiver action plan
- Inquire about caregiver's biggest fear or concern
- Ask if caregiver has additional support already in place
- Encourage caregiver to ask questions of healthcare team and to be proactive
- Offer assistance with connecting to community resources and scheduling provider follow up appointments

Caregiver Type	Caregiver Need (what this type needs but may not realize)	Caregiver Preferences (what this type is drawn to and receptive of)
Manager	• To assess and integrate most fitting approach to care, rather than the first available	• Information on disease • Care planning with clear support markers from providers • Description of treatment, common reactions
Carrier	• To assess and integrate information about ways to distribute caregiving labors	• Directions for hands on care • Regular contact with providers to confirm caregiving labors and execution • Strategies for monitoring physical, social, and cognitive changes in the care receiver
Partner	• To assess and integrate information that can clarify care plan and its execution	• Information on disease • Physical, social, and cognitive changes for the patient • Practical actions to support care recipient across a range of needs (biopsychosocial)
Lone	• To assess and integrate information that surpasses biomedical needs	• Opportunities and options for care beyond current care plan • Care approaches to delay disease processes • Medical resources that may be heavily driven by research

© Comfort Communication Project

assess information that will or will not ultimately be useful. This domain helps the caregiver distinguish appropriate health systems resources for optimal patient care. Learning about caregiver understanding of disease process and intent of treatment is central to this domain. Gaining an understanding of the caregiver's preferred ways to learn and use new information (e.g., print, online, and text messaging) will serve to help the provider best partner with the caregiver in information use.

Partnering with the Caregiver

In this domain, the essential dynamic of connecting with and attending to the caregiver is the focus. Here, we prioritize the caregiver as a second-order patient and task the provider to obtain information from and create information with the caregiver. Knowledge shared with caregiver will become part of charting to inform vital health information for provider teams (Table 9.3).

Finding Support

This domain invites the provider to actuate resources and help for the caregiver, specific to their greatest challenges (Table 9.4). Appraising opportunities and acceptability for the caregiver to accept or decline support (social, emotional, psychological, respite, peer, provider, community-based services, spiritual/religious) is essential to finding support to aid them in the journey of caregiving. Knowing about caregiver support and actually finding tailored support for a specific caregiver are two different tasks.

Talking with the Caregiver

Communicating with the caregiver is a skill that can be developed, practiced, and delivered in a way that will result in improved patient care, as well as caregiver outcomes. Defining topic areas for communication is an important first step and can be informed by learning about the type of caregiver you are with (Table 9.5). Understanding some aspects of that caregiver's relationship to the care recipient is really essential in engaging the caregiver.

Planning for Caregiver Self-Care

Dedicated efforts to support the health and well-being of the caregiver is the focus of this domain (Table 9.6). The caregiver types each regard self-care with different importance, yet we know that self-care is essential to caregiver health, longevity, and performance for the care recipient. Acknowledging burnout and caregiver burden is central to this communication. Also learning about the caregiver's

Table 9.3 PARTNERING WITH THE CAREGIVER

Recommended Provider Strategies
- Learn about caregiver's social, spiritual and cultural beliefs and behaviors
- Formulate open ended questions for the caregiver
- Identify caregiver strengths (i.e., resilience, resources, adaptability) and areas of limitation (i.e. logistic concerns, current psychological or family issues)
- Prioritize the needs and concerns of caregiver
- Track caregiver needs and concerns across time points
- Invite caregiver engagement (e.g., audio recording, notes, planning for visits)
- Collaborate with other providers on the plan of care and additional support needed
- Share a list of provider numbers and resources specific to that caregiver/care recipient case

Caregiver Type	*Caregiver Need* (what this type needs but may not realize it)	*Caregiver Preferences* (what this type is drawn to and receptive of)
Manager	• To partner with provider to best achieve credible and most appropriate care plan for care recipient	• Communication about care planning • Communication about care execution • Attention to action-oriented work that can be achieved and coordinated by caregiver
Carrier	• To partner with provider to best achieve support for caregiving choices in the present and across the disease path	• Opportunity to share concerns and worries with provider • Receiving monitored support from provider about caregiving concerns and worries • Exchanging ideas about available resources found outside of family network
Partner	• To partner with provider to best achieve coherent caregiving and planning throughout caregiving network	• Coordination of caregiving plan across caregiving network • Integration of care recipient into caregiving plan • Inclusion of caregiver limitations and resources in communication
Lone	• To partner with provider to best achieve quality patient care in mental, social, and emotional health	• Communication about care planning that includes shared ideas and challenges • Reliance on close communication with provider about decisions and goals about care • Opportunities to share about caregiving needs and worries with provider and care recipient

© Comfort Communication Project

Table 9.4 FINDING SUPPORT

Recommended Provider Strategies
- Identify and evaluate the caregiver's current support system (e.g., Caregiver Distress Screener)
- Ask caregiver if they would like to include support system in discussions, appointments, etc.
- Inquire about specific forms of support and what that caregiver appraises as acceptable forms of support (e.g., checklist of support opportunities, verbalized ideas of support)
- Assist caregiver to develop a comprehensive support list (i.e. transportation services, notary, support groups, case management, caregiver services, etc.)
- Offer to assist caregiver with linkage to support services
- Anticipate and promptly respond to signs that caregiver help may be needed (e.g., anxiety, exhaustion, withdrawal, weight change)
- Provide opportunities for the caregiver to share about their work as caregiver

Caregiver Type	*Caregiver Need* (what this type needs but may not realize it)	*Caregiver Preferences* (what this type is drawn to and receptive of)
Manager	• To receive a range of resources that can be implemented and disseminated by the caregiver to provide time away	• Engaging support in the form of tasks and goals • Identification of tasks for others in family network • Incorporation of trusted support resources into regimen of care plans
Carrier	• To receive supportive care focused on caregiver burden, specifically outside of the construct of family	• Open to receiving support sources outside of family structure and care recipient • Open to receiving care specific to self • Receptive to specific caregiving task training and planning
Partner	• To receive a range of support that can be used across caregiving network to help establish more coherence in care plan	• Support that will impact the care recipient • Eager to learn about and incorporate resources across caregiving network • Support that can offer coherence to day-to-day care plan and understanding of disease process
Lone	• To receive psychosocial support	• Support resources that can be engaged by the dyad of caregiver/care recipient • Support that addresses physical impact of disease process in creative ways • Process support options in relationship with providers (the primary network for the Lone)

© Comfort Communication Project

Table 9.5 TALKING WITH THE CAREGIVER

Recommended Provider Strategies
- Learn caregiver's language preference or desire for language assistance
- Ask what the caregiver already knows about the disease process
- Invite the caregiver's personal attitudes and values that relate to the care recipient
- Present opportunities for conversations about the greatest concerns for the caregiver
- Speak in plain language
- Chunk and check information and incorporate teach back
- Avoid use of acronyms, idioms, and abbreviations
- Provide open and honest information with the caregiver
- Engage the caregiver about cultural, religious, and spiritual preferences
- Allow time to listen to the caregiver
- Discuss and describe palliative care

Caregiver Type	Caregiver Need (what this type needs but may not realize it)	Caregiver Preferences (what this type is drawn to and receptive of)
Manager	• To communicate with provider about the impact of caregiving on their own life	• Discussion of treatment plan • Incorporation of medical language and ideas • Deflection of caregiver burden in favor of care recipient needs
Carrier	• To communicate about greatest concerns/worries about caregiving and create an action plan to address them/cope	• Reviewing caregiving choices • Sharing caregiving anxieties • Reluctance to distribute caregiving labors across family network
Partner	• To communicate various perspectives and needs of the caregiving network into care plans—short and long term.	• Engages the aspect of caregiving work with which they are familiar rather than overall care needs • Integrates provider ideas and concerns into caregiving labors • Centers the care receiver's needs in any interaction
Lone	• To build a trusted partnership with provider in light of a minimal or non-existent family network	• Focus on the physical aspects of care • Incorporates the burden on the caregiver/care recipient dyad • Avoids topics addressing caregiver needs

© Comfort Communication Project

Table 9.6 PLANNING FOR CAREGIVER SELF-CARE

Recommended Provider Strategies
- Evaluate the caregiver's current self-care habits (e.g., food, sleep, medical care, mental healthcare, support network)
- Assist to create a plan for caregiver self-care (e.g., stress reduction practices, morning walk with friends, scheduled time off without guilt)
- Assess caregiver self-care actions and needs regularly
- Inquire about specific forms of self-care and what the caregiver views as acceptable and possible
- Inquire about caregiver's future plans as care recipient's needs change
- Share suggestions and offer information on additional community resources
- Offer to connect with other caregivers in community
- Provide contact information for caregiver to reach out if having difficulty with role and responsibilities, emotions such as anger, guilt, grief or frustration

Caregiver Type	*Caregiver Need* (what this type needs but may not realize it)	*Caregiver Preferences* (what this type is drawn to and receptive of)
Manager	• To experience self-care with special emphasis on mental and spiritual healthcare.	• Engaging self-care in the form of doing things for others • Coordination of care recipient's care to create an opportunity for self-care • Involvement in activity and action over stillness and relaxation
Carrier	• To experience self-care across physical, mental, spiritual, and psychological domains.	• Guided by support of providers to receive self-care • Finding help outside of family structure or family knowledge • Receptive to identified self-care, but deterred by having to invest time and energy in finding it
Partner	• To receive a range of support that can be used across caregiving network to help establish more coherence in care plan	• Receptive to self-care that may also help others in the caregiving network • Receptive to self-care that may also help the care receiver • Receptive to new and previously unknown opportunities
Lone	• To experience self-care with special emphasis on physical and mental healthcare.	• Desires self-care but is reticent to leave care recipient • Avoids planning and executing self-care in order to be available to care recipient, as they function closely as a dyad • Focuses on next "fire" for care recipient

© Comfort Communication Project

self-care abilities will help guide conversations about planning for burnout intervention. Without provider support, it is difficult for some caregivers to give themselves permission to take time and care for themselves.

FUTURE RESEARCH

As we have presented the typology to interdisciplinary audiences of healthcare providers and researchers over the last decade, we have been commonly asked about the rigidity of the typology. Can an individual actually be a blend of two types? Is it possible for an individual to move from one type to another? Essentially, we do not believe that caregivers change their type if their family system is unchanged; but we do believe that all caregivers can learn new communication and health literacy skills for communication about chronic illness.

Throughout this volume we have demonstrated that family members communicate in recognizably patterned ways (i.e., the types), historically constructed through family hierarchy/role, genetic propensity, cultural background, etc. The goal of future research is not to identify the type or types of caregivers most facilitative to good patient outcomes, but rather it will investigate how best to support *each* type in the caregiving journey by facilitating open awareness and communication. For example, we do not expect that the Carrier caregiver will develop a sharp skill set for delegating like the Manager caregiver, but we do hope that we can provide caregiver support and education to the Carrier caregiver to learn to ask for help. The communication pattern established between care recipient and caregiver is patterned and essentially fixed; it is the topic and context of communication where new skills can be developed to improve the caregiving experience and thus improve patient and caregiver outcomes.

To expand our understanding of the typology, we see potential connections and explorations needed in the following areas:

- The influence of care recipient's communication patterns on caregiver type (e.g., what impact does patient communication skill training have on caregiver types?)
- The influence of a healthcare provider's tailored approach on caregiver type communication (e.g., what impact do specific communication techniques have on caregiver types?)
- How a caregiver's prior caregiving experience may influence caregiving
- Address whether caregiver types vary in terms of resilience, social support needs, and use and function of social support systems
- How a caregiver's type impacts bereavement
- The quality and quantity of patient discussion about end-of-life wishes between caregiver types
- Address how different caregiver types are related to care recipient's satisfaction with caregiving and overall quality of life
- Preferences for where to deliver end-of-life care among caregiver types

- Advance care planning discussions between care recipient and caregiver types
- Dyadic caregiving dynamics and care outcomes
- The role of intersectional variables such as gender, culture, social determinants, religion/spirituality, and age on caregiver types, interventions, and their outcomes.

CONCLUSION

A well-established foundational tenet of palliative care is that healthcare providers should care for the patient and family caregiver unit together, as one comprehensive team (National Consensus Project for Quality Palliative Care, 2018). As shared throughout the chapter narratives, the reality is that family caregivers are often left alone to fend for themselves on the sideline. They share the experience of living with the uncertainty of chronic illness (Reigada et al., 2015). Caregivers are a population at risk who continually express feelings of exclusion, frustration, neglect, fear, and overwhelming distress.

Research in the caregiving literature reports that system level factors contribute to caregiver difficulty, specifically with accessing and navigating for healthcare services, communicating about health, and obtaining support and resources (Fields et al., 2018). In palliative care, limited health literacy is associated with poor pain management, medication errors, nonadherence to the proposed treatment plan (Wittenberg et al., 2015) and uncertainty with decision-making when completing advanced directives (Sudore et al., 2018). These experiences and implications can be improved with enhanced health literacy and effective communication.

Existing family patterns, experiences, relationships, roles, and expectations collectively contribute to the caregiving experience. It is our hope that the provision of the FCCT will assist healthcare providers in lessening caregiver burden and provide caregiver communication and health literacy interventions that support, guide. and educate each caregiver type through their caregiving journey.

We present this volume to reconsider the essential role of caregiving across the life cycle, re-evaluate the impact of caregiving on the care recipient and caregiver, and recognize the complexity of family caregiving and the vital need to integrate caregivers as a crucial member of the healthcare team. This is our call, therefore, to truly *care for the family caregiver*, the backbone of our nation's long-term care system.

REFERENCES

Bangerter, L. R., Griffin, J. M., Zarit, S. H., & Havyer, R. (2019). Measuring the needs of family caregivers of people with dementia: An assessment of current methodological strategies and key recommendations. *Journal of Applied Gerontology, 38*(9), 1304–1318. https://doi.org/10.1177/0733464817705959

Behforouz, H. L., Drain, P. K., & Rhatigan, J. J. (2014). Rethinking the social history. *New England Journal of Medicine, 317*(14), 1277–9. doi: 10.1056/NEJMp1404846.

Bell, J. F., Whitney, R. L., & Young, H. M. (2019). Family caregiving in serious illness in the United States: Recommendations to support an invisible workforce. *Journal of American Geriatrics Society, 67*(S2), S451–S456. https://doi.org/10.1111/jgs.15820

Bennett, N. M., Brown, M. T., Green, T., Hall, L. L., & Winkler, A. M. (2018). Addressing social determinants of health (SDOH): Beyond the clinic walls. *American Medical Association.* https://edhub.ama-assn.org/steps-forward/module/2702762

Bucknall, T. K., Hutchinson, A. M., Botti, M., McTier, L., Rawson, H., Hitch, D., . . . Chaboyer, W. (2020). Engaging patients and families in communication across transitions of care: An integrative review. *Patient and Education Counseling.* https://doi.org/10.1016/j.pec.2020.01.017

Campione, J. R., & Zebrak, K. A. (2020). Predictors of unmet need among informal caregivers. *Journal of Gerontology, Series B: Psychological Sciences and Social Sciences.* https://doi.org/10.1093/geronb/gbz165

Chappell, R. Y. (2016). Incentivizing patient choices: The ethics of inclusive shared savings. *Bioethics,30*(8), 597–600. https://doi.org/10.1111/bioe.12267

Fields, B., Rodakowski, J., Everette, J. A., & Beach, S. (2018). Caregiver health literacy predicting healthcare communication and system navigation difficulty. *American Psychological Association, 36*(4), 482–492. https://doi.org/10.1037/fsh0000368

Gerain, P., & Zech, E. (2019). Informal caregiver burnout? Development of a theoretical framework to understand the impact of caregiving. *Frontiers in Psychology, 10*, 1748. https://doi.org/10.3389/fpsyg.2019.01748

Gonella, S., Campagna, S., Basso, I., De Marinis, M. G., & Di Giulio, P. (2019, December). Mechanisms by which end-of-life communication influences palliative-oriented care in nursing homes: A scoping review. *Patient & Education Counseling, 102*(12), 2134–2144. https://doi.org/10.1016/j.pec.2019.06.018

Kokorelias, K. M., Gignac, M. A. M., Naglie, G., & Cameron, J. I. (2019). Towards a universal model of family centered care: A scoping review. *BMC Health Services Research, 19*(1), 564. https://doi.org/10.1186/s12913-019-4394-5

Logan, R. A., Wong, W. F., Villaire, M., Daus, G., Parnell, T. A., Willis, E., & Paasche-Orlow, M. (2015). Health literacy: A necessary element for achieving health equity (Discussion paper). *National Academy of Medicine.* Retrieved from https://nam.edu/perspectives-2015-health-literacy-a-necessary-element-for-achieving-health-equity/

National Consensus Project for Quality Palliative Care. (2018). *Clinical practice guidelines for quality palliative care.* https://www.nationalcoalitionhpc.org/ncp

Parker, R. M., & Ratzan, S. (2019). Re-enforce, not re-define health literacy-moving forward with health literacy 2.0. *Journal of Health Communication, 24*(12), 923–925. https://doi.org/10.1080/10810730.2019.1691292

Reigada, C., Pais-Ribeiro, J., Novellas, A., & Gonçalves, E. (2015). The caregiver role in palliative care: A systematic review of the literature. *Health Care Current Reviews, 3*(2), 143. https://doi.org/10.4172/2375-4273.1000143

Rowlands, G., Shaw, A., Jaswal, S., Smith, S., & Harpham, T. (2017). Health literacy and the social determinants of health: A qualitative model from adult learners. *Health Promotion International, 32*(1), 130–138. doi: 10.1093/heapro/dav093

Sudore, R., Schillinger, D., Katen, M., Shi, Y., Boscardin, J., Osua, S., & Barnes, D. (2018). Engaging diverse English and Spanish speaking older adults in advance care planning. *JAMA Internal Medicine,* 178, 1616–1625. https://doi.org/10.1001/jamainternmed.2018.4657

Thomas, C., Turner, M., Payne, S., Milligan, C., Brearley, S., Seamark, D., . . . Blake, S. (2018). Family carers' experiences of coping with the deaths of adults in home settings: A narrative analysis of carers' relevant background worries. *Palliative Medicine, 32*(5), 950–959. https://doi.org/10.1177/0269216318757134

Wittenberg, E., Goldsmith, J., Ferrell, B., & Platt, C. S. (2015). Enhancing communication related to symptom management through plain language: A brief report. *Journal of Pain & Symptom Management, 50*(5), 707–711. https://doi.org/10.1016/j.jpainsymman.2015.06.007

Zavagli, V., Raccichini, M., Ercolani, G., Franchini, L., Varani, S., & Pannuti, R. (2019). Care for carers: An investigation on family caregivers' needs, tasks, and experiences. *Translational Medicine UniSa, 19,* 54–59. https://www.ncbi.nlm.nih.gov/pubmed/31360668

Tables, figures and boxes are indicated by *t, f* and *b* following the page number